# The Parent
# CONNECTION

# The Parent
# CONNECTION

## Susan Boe

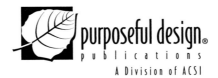
purposeful design.
p u b l i c a t i o n s
A Division of ACSI

Purposeful Design Publications is the publishing division of the Association of Christian Schools International (ACSI) and is committed to the ministry of Christian school education, to enable Christian educators and schools worldwide to effectively prepare students for life. As the publisher of textbooks, trade books, and other educational resources within ACSI, Purposeful Design Publications strives to produce biblically sound materials that reflect Christian scholarship and stewardship and that address the identified needs of Christian schools around the world.

References to books, computer software, and other ancillary resources in this series are not endorsements by ACSI. These materials were selected to provide teachers with additional resources appropriate to the concepts being taught and to promote student understanding and enjoyment.

Printed in the United States of America
16                                        5 6 7

Boe, Susan
  *The parent connection: A health education resource for parents of teens*
  Second edition
  Total Health series
  ISBN 978-1-58331-235-3   Catalog #7610

Purposeful Design Publications
*A Division of ACSI*
PO Box 65130 • Colorado Springs, CO 80962-5130
Customer Service: 800-367-0798 • www.acsi.org

# -The Parent
# CONNECTION

*continued*

# Introduction

## A Unique Opportunity

Did you know that you are about to make history? *The Parent Connection* is the first book of its kind. It brings health education into the home. It is a valuable tool to help parents talk with their teens about health-related issues.

Whether in school or in the home, a health course is a totally unique opportunity for Christian young people to be trained in the making of wise choices. No other course in the entire school curriculum directly addresses the teen issues that students are personally experiencing at the same time as they are learning about them. Math class doesn't address a teen's present hormonal changes. Reading a textbook on American History might be interesting, but it doesn't train a teen not to drink alcohol or take drugs. English class may instruct teens on proper spelling and grammar, but it doesn't help a student deal with relationships with family or friends. The fact that teens are actually living the same topics that they are studying raises their interest level and makes them extremely receptive to positive input about these vital issues in their lives.

Wouldn't it be great if the consequences of our teens' choices were low-risk and uncomplicated? As we all know, they aren't. The choices which face our teens today are more complex and involve much higher stakes. Many are even life-threatening. One of the major reasons why teen decisions today are so much more complex than several years ago is because each major area of their life and their surrounding culture is undergoing tumultuous changes. Along with *every* change, there are more options presented to them. Teens desire more and more independence with which to make their own choices. Even at the age of nine, my son Steven is seeking independence. The choices he faces at his age such as where to ride his bike, what friend to play with, or what toy to share do not compare to the decisions that face teenagers. Although teen choices are very different they can be categorized into four general areas: physical choices, mental choices, social choices, and spiritual choices. These are the four main unit divisions of the *Total Health* curriculum (see "Using *The Parent Connection* Alongside the *Total Health* School Curriculum") that correspond with this Parent Manual.

Regarding their physical choices, teens no longer run to their parents every time they get hurt or don't feel well. Moreover, their bodies are experiencing the hormonal changes that come with adolescence. They are confronted with loaded questions and contradictory messages from their surrounding culture. Mentally, teens do not automatically come to Mom or Dad to talk about what makes them feel "sad." Instead, they talk with their peers and may begin to shape their ideals apart from home. Socially, they begin to get a taste of an "unchaperoned" life and the independence that comes with a driver's license. Spiritually, teens are searching for a meaning to their existence. They are beginning to make the personal choices that will lead them to a powerful relationship with God through a personal ownership of their faith.

## The Faith Perspective

Upon seeing so many options for teens with such serious implications, some parents develop a fear perspective toward the teenage years. In an effort to guard and protect their teens against making any wrong choices that could harm them, parents can become defensive, demanding, rigid, and legalistic.

> When parents try to lay down rules without first establishing a real relationship with their children, the natural result will be rebellion. Sometimes it will be outward rebellion that is easy to spot in the child's actions, but just as often it can be an inward rebellion, where the child appears to be obedient but is nursing all kinds of grudges and hangups, along with an unhealthy self-image and poor self-esteem.[1]

Although their motive is good, the overall result is usually disastrous. Put simply, the teens rebel. Josh McDowell reminds us as parents:

Rules without relationship lead to rebellion.[2]

Because the fear perspective of parenting is overprotective, it does not prepare the teen to make real choices based upon personal convictions.

> Nothing intimidates us quite like our responsibilities as parents. The thought that our inadequacies could cause the permanent downfall of our children can rob us of the joy of parenthood. By having a strategy for developing our children's character, we release our spirits from the bondage of fear.[3]

But what happens all too often is that the parent-teen relationship of trust developed at home is not strong enough to keep young people away from the temptations of our culture. *The Parent Connection* is an excellent tool which helps parents develop that relationship of trust with their teen.

*When I began to hear very personal, questions, comments, and admissions from my students* in class, I knew that my old way of teaching health was just not going to work anymore. The main reason that it wasn't going to be adequate to prepare teens for their futures was that my old style of teaching was subconsciously based on a perspective of fear — fear that teens would fall away from the Lord if given much freedom at all. Consequently, I centered my teaching on lecturing and note taking and avoided their hard and embarrassing questions. I did not get good results. Once I changed my perspective, however, I began to see much better results. I found that I was developing a closer relationship with my students because of the discussions we were having in class and privately. I was seeing lives changed as students began to process decisions for themselves, hear honest answers, and see God as a loving and practical God.

My new faith perspective helped me to see the entire teenage journey as an essential part of God's preordained plan of developing young people into Christian adults who are trained (rather than forced) to make wise choices of their own. The faith perspective toward health education is based on the gradual giving of privileges based on a relationship of trust, the freedom to ask hard and embarrassing questions, and the right to form personal opinions — even when those opinions aren't exactly what others believe. This dialogue method is the same kind of method that we use in The Parent Connection. The Parent Connection helps to prepare teens for the real world of decision-making. As you dive into this approach, be prepared; you will learn much about your teen, your family, and yourself!

# How to Use This Resource Most Successfully

There are several factors that will determine the success of this method. One suggestion is that, to the best of your ability, your teen should not know you are using *The Parent Connection*. This book is your own private health resource and communication tool. Your interaction with your teen(s) will be the most effective the more it is on a casual, natural, everyday level. If teens feel that their parents are just reading to them out of another "textbook," rather than sharing genuinely out of their own true life experiences, they will tend not to respond or interact. Teaching our teens in the course of normal everyday activities is just what the Bible is referring to when it says, "You shall teach these laws to your children when you sit in your house, when you take a walk along the road, when you go to bed, and when you get up in the morning." (Deuteronomy 11:19)

It's never too late to begin to develop better lines of communication with your teen. *The Parent Connection* will be one tool that will help you to "connect" with your young adult.

As you read *The Parent Connection*, please note that the use of his/her are written interchangeably.

This is how to use it:

- Take a brief tour. Glance through *The Parent Connection* to get an overview of its overall format.

- If using the *Total Health* curriculum, note the subjects your teen will be covering in each unit of the *Total Health* student text. This would be a good time to contact the health teacher to gather information on what is being taught. *The Parent Connection* lists the page numbers that correspond to those subjects covered in the student text. (See Appendix A.)

- Identify the issues. To the best of your knowledge, decide what specific issue(s) your teen is personally facing. Look over the subjects that are listed in *The Parent Connection*. (If you aren't sure, just stick to the class assignment topics you can get from the teacher or your child). The goal is for you and your teen to be able to casually and naturally interact. This will open up health issues for discussion between you and your teen as he is doing his *Total Health* homework.

- Choose the issues. Write down the subject(s) that best relates to you and/ or your teen's personal situation. You may find issues that only interest you.

- Connect with the issues. Turn to that specific teen issue in *The Parent Connection* and follow the numbered steps:

    1. Know the Causes: the overview you may need to adequately prepare you for the issue.
    2. Observe Your Teen: the challenge of being honest about yourself and your teen.
    3. Talk with Your Teen: the means to start relevant conversations with your teen(s) — asking him sincere questions and listening respectfully to his responses.
    4. Take Action: the steps to make it all happen; by you caring enough to take action.
    5. Pause to Reflect: the reflection questions to help you check your "connecting" progress.

- Consider further resources. Select the sources you may need to get further help or insight to help your teenager.

## Using *The Parent Connection* Alongside the *Total Health* School Curriculum

### *(See Appendix A)*

Because there was a lack of middle school and high school Christian health curriculum until recently, the old health curriculum approach was either not to use a health textbook, to use a secular textbook, or to use a secular textbook and avoid objectionable pages. Generally speaking, Health class has been on the bottom of the priority list in the Christian school and home school curriculum. The *Total Health* method, on the other hand, is unique. It places a biblical emphasis on the importance of health education. It addresses all relevant issues in a balanced, modest, and general way. It also provides for the students an opportunity for discussion in a controlled environment. *Total Health* provides both school and parent with a definite strategy of protecting teens from unnecessary risks as they personalize their Christian faith and ethics.

The benefit to you of having your teen in a *Total Health* class with a trained health teacher who uses our guided discussion methods, is that you gain an extra pair of eyes and ears through which you can be made aware of health issues that concern your teenager.

The *Total Health* teacher is trained to impart biblical values as "teachable moments" occur in the classroom. One day a rather shocking teachable moment surprised me. As I was teaching on the subject of nutrition, one of the female students in my health class made the following statement about women's sexuality: "It's just not fair. Why is everything so hard for a woman? I heard that it hurts to have intercourse; it hurts to have a baby; it hurts to breast feed; and it hurts when we get our period. This is just not fair!"

When I heard these words, I realized that I had to be very careful in how I responded. The classroom of girls was silent; all eyes were on me. I knew that this girl was not just seeking attention through her comment; she was totally serious.

These "yellow-flag" stories occurred quite frequently in my health class. They indicated to me that parents needed to become aware of the concerns facing their teenager. I also realized that *every* parent of a teen in my class probably wished they had a secret audio tape of all of our class discussions. It was at this point that I began to see how much parents needed a communication tool to build a bridge between themselves, their teen, and the health issues that they were experiencing. Thus, *The Parent Connection*.

The process is that simple. So, let's get started. It's now time to "connect" with your teen!

# PHYSICAL HEALTH

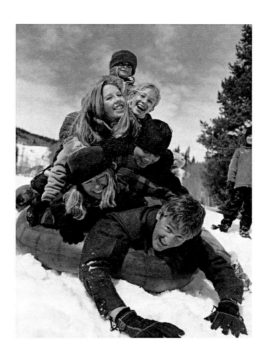

*Your body is the house in which you live. By analogy, it is just like the building in which you make your home. Your home needs, at the very least, periodical attention, otherwise the roof may leak, the plumbing may get out of order and clog up, termites may drill through the floors and the walls, and other innumerable causes of deterioration may make their appearance. Such is the case with your physical body. Every function and activity of your system, day and night, physical, mental, and spiritual, is dependent on the attention you give it. [4]*

# Nutrition Battles

*If you do not smoke or drink excessively, your diet can influence your long-term health prospects more than any other action you might take.*[5]

Several factors influence the food choices teens make: culture, the people they admire or respect (those Pepsi® commercials can do it!), the school, the media, and the food choices of friends. During the early years through preadolescence, the most powerful influence on a child's health behavior is the family. Upon entering adolescence, however, society, peers, and a teen's self-image begin to have a stronger influence upon his food habits. If you want to begin to change the eating habits of your teen, first discover the cause of the poor eating habit. Once the source is found, a poor habit can be relearned and become a positive habit.

## *1* Know the Causes

I'm aware that most of a child's eating habits are established at an early age and by the influence of the home. As a child matures, his peers and the media begin to play more of a role in his food choices. A basic fact of nutrition is that the more a person feeds the body healthy food, the more the body craves healthy food. Unfortunately, the converse is also true. The more a person feeds the body unhealthy (junk) food, the more the body craves that which is unhealthy.

## 2 Observe Your Teen

Can you recognize any of the following that may be influencing your teen's eating habits?

- A low self-esteem causing her to eat too much? Yes / No / I don't know

- A low self-esteem causing her to eat too little? Yes / No / I don't know

- A fast-paced schedule in which he is too busy to eat? Yes / No / I don't know

- What meals might he miss on a regular basis?
     Breakfast? Lunch?     Dinner?

- A fast-paced schedule causing him to eat unhealthily? Yes / No / I don't know

- Any negative family eating patterns, e.g., late night snacks, in-between meal snacks, high fat snacks? Yes / No / I don't know

- Fast food or restaurant dining instead of eating at home? Yes (if yes, how often?) / No / I don't know

- Family eating meals together? Yes / No / I don't know

- You can figure the percentage of meals that your teen eats with the family per week by following the formula below. It assumes that the number of meals the average person consumes per week is 21 (7 days per week x 3 meals per day = 21 meals per week).

  A.  The number of meals that your teen eats with the family per week is ____.

  B.  Divide A (above) by 21. This will give you the percentage of meals that your teen eats with your family each week.

If your teen is struggling with making healthy food choices, try to find out if he is open to change by using the Conversation Starters listed below. If he is open, you have half of the battle won! If your teen is absolutely closed to making changes, you may need to make changes so slowly that he doesn't notice. For example, you might substitute 1% milk for the 2% your family drinks. The example you and the family set in your own eating habits will help your teen develop new healthy ones.

The most positive changes should begin in the home. The key is to shoot for lifelong changes rather than only immediate results.

## 3 Talk with Your Teen

It's most natural to discuss food issues while in the kitchen fixing a meal or while your teen is preparing a snack. Remember, this is not a time to judge what or how much they are eating at the moment but rather to use it as a springboard to open up discussion about the larger issues of general health, the importance of nutrition for teenagers, nutrition and exercise, causes of tiredness, media-created food images, low self-esteem, etc. After reading all of the following questions, choose which ones would be the most effective ways for you to use to begin a casual conversation with your teen. Remember that your purpose is to get your teen to open up — not shut down as a result of you dominating the conversation.

- *"If you were stranded on an island but could only have one food choice, what would you pick? Why?"*

- *"What do you think is the greatest influence on your food choices? Why?"*

- *"Did you know that statistics show that teenagers have very poor eating habits? Why do you think that is?"*

- *"I heard that every minute three Americans have a heart attack. Why do you think Americans are so prone to heart disease? Do you think that it is stress-related? Do you think that it may be diet-related?"*

- *"When you're out on your own, you'll be more responsible for your own cooking and grocery shopping. How would you change the way we have done things for the family? What have you learned from us at home that will help you when you are on your own? Would you cook like we do for your family if you get married someday?"*

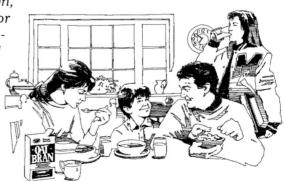

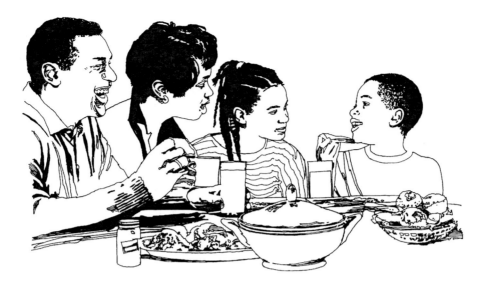

- *"Check out the dinner we are having tonight. How does it rate taste-wise? What do you think would make it a healthier meal?"*

- *"Have you noticed how soda pop is such a popular drink? Just out of curiosity, do you think teens drink more soda pop than adults? Why or why not? How many overweight people have you seen drinking diet pop? (A lot, probably!) If diet pop truly helps a person lose weight, why are so many people still overweight who drink it? I read that diet soda can actually make you gain weight because the sodium that it contains causes the body to retain water. I also read that all artificial sweeteners trick your body so that it's unable to metabolize fat properly. Diet pop also depletes the body of essential minerals. Have you personally experienced any health benefits from drinking pop? I've been thinking about cutting down on my own soda intake. If I make an effort to really try, would you help remind me? Do you want to try to cut down with me?"*

- *"I understand you've been working on a food journal. Can you explain how it works? I would also like to keep a food journal while you're doing yours. Let's work on it together, OK?"*

- *"We've been so busy lately, that I feel like our good eating habits are being challenged. What do you think that we can do to slow down and make time for eating more meals as a family each week?"*

**Take Action**

When making observations and suggestions concerning your teen's eating habits, it's very common for a parent to want to see immediate changes. The most beneficial kinds of eating changes, however, are not temporary ones. The best changes are adjustments in daily eating habits based upon personal convictions. These will stay with your teen throughout his life. Remember that the ultimate goal is a healthy lifestyle not just temporary changes.

### My Daily Food Journal

| | Sun. | Mon. | Tues. | Wed. | Thurs. | Fri. | Sat. |
|---|---|---|---|---|---|---|---|
| **Date:** | | | | | | | |
| Breakfast | | | | | | | |
| Snack | | | | | | | |
| Lunch | | | | | | | |
| Snack | | | | | | | |
| Dinner | | | | | | | |
| Snack | | | | | | | |
| **Comments:** | | | | | | | |

❑ **Food Journal:**

Encourage the food journal as it is assigned in class. Ask your teen to show you how it works and do one along with her. At the end of each week, get together with your teen and compare journals. Share together about the eating habits that each of you have. After your teen sees that you are willing to admit your own food related weaknesses, she will be more willing to open up about her own needs. You'll find it to be a great strength and bonding experience for both of you. If you are successful at this, you may want to try suggesting that every family member keep a food journal.

❏ **Meal Planning for Extra Credit:**

Ask your teen's health teacher if your child could get extra credit for planning and cooking one meal a week. If acceptable to the teacher, have your teen help you plan the entire meal from main entrée to dessert, and then go with you to the store to shop for the food or, go to the store for himself. He must cook the complete meal, and then evaluate it for cost-efficiency, taste, and good nutrition. Finally, you write an evaluation of the meal and send it to the teacher for credit.

❏ **Brainstorming Session:**

What family patterns can you change that will help your teen change some poor eating habits? Have a brainstorming session some night during dinner about this.

---

## *Self-Inventory of Family Patterns*

Eating patterns begin with the family and help shape your future eating habits.

1. What do I notice about my family's attitude toward food?

2. Any specific family eating habits? (positive and/or negative)

3. What do I notice about my family's attitude toward exercise?

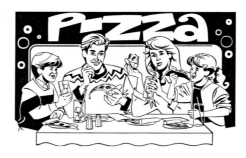

4. How does my family handle stress?

5. Does my family eat out at restaurants or fast food restaurants regularly? How often?

6. How often does my family eat meals together?

7. Do I notice anyone in my family eating breakfast regularly? Do I eat breakfast regularly?

---

❏ **Substitution Rather than Elimination:**
Instead of making drastic changes and immediately eliminating everyone's favorite foods, begin to substitute slightly lower-fat snacks for higher-fat snacks around the house. E.g., use pretzels instead of potato chips or chips that are low in fat and/or low in salt. Every once in a while, buy their favorite snack so they don't think you have gone "purist." Substitute 1% milk for 2%. Keep the 2% carton (clean it out well) and add 1% milk. If they don't notice the difference, start buying 1%. Substitution rather than elimination can bring gradual eating changes into your teen's life. If the changes are gradual, they are more likely to stick. If your teen responds positively to all of your gradual changes, you can go ahead and make larger ones.

❏ **Meal Preparation:**
Involve your children, on a regular or rotational basis, in the planning and cooking of meals. To add motivation, let them choose their own favorite meal (within reason).

❏ **Cookbook Evaluation:**
Sit down and go through your cookbooks. Evaluate them according to your understanding of nutritional values. Look for low-fat, low-sugar, low-salt, stone-ground whole wheat flour recipes. If you find that there are not enough "healthy ideas" to keep you motivated, take your teen with you to a local health food store or bookstore and have him help you pick out a few new books that fit your criteria.

# *5* **Pause to Reflect**

After you finish the appropriate Action Steps, complete this evaluation to see how the chapter worked for you.

● How well did you "connect" with your teen on this issue?

Not very well        Fairly well        Very well

● How well did the Conversation Starters work with getting your teen to open up?        Not very well        Fairly well        Very well

● What did you discover about your teen that you did not know before?

- What did you learn about your teen's reason(s) for eating the way he does?


- What did you find out about your family as a result of this material?


- What did this section teach you about yourself?


- How successful were the Action Steps in your situation?

  Not successful          Very successful          Don't know/can't tell yet

- Record any further insights, questions, or comments concerning food choices and your teen below:


## Further Resources

*Eat Well, Live Well,* Pamela Smith, (Creation House, 1992).

*Food For Life,* Pamela Smith, (Creation House, 1994).

*Healthy Living in a Toxic World,* Cynthia Fincher Ph.D. (Pinon Press, 1996).

*Juicing For Life: A Guide to the Benefits of Fresh Fruit and Vegetable Juicing,* Cherie Calbom and Maureen Keane, (Avery Publishing Group, 1992).

*The Natural Way To Vibrant Health,* Dr. N.W. Walker, (Norwalk Press, 1972).

# Eating Disorders
## Anorexia, Bulimia, and Overeating

Later that Christmas night, after my parents had gone to bed, I quietly snuck back to the kitchen, determined to taste everything I'd missed. I grabbed a roll, dipped it into the gravy boat, and crammed it into my mouth. Then I ate some stuffing. Then a bite of a vegetable casserole. Next, some pecans off the pie. Suddenly, I realized I'd gone too far. In two minutes I had destroyed an all-day effort to avoid eating. Well, no need to get depressed. I might as well eat my fill of everything now. I'll just have to get rid of it later. I knew how. I'd done it dozens of times before.

Mindlessly, I began shoveling handfuls of food into my mouth. I devoured huge amounts of leftovers from Christmas dinner, breakfast, and even from days before. My distended stomach ached — I must have looked six months pregnant. My food frenzy began to slow down when I could no longer walk without bending over. Once in the bathroom, I completed the now familiar ritual I'd begun this time with that first bite of turkey. I forced my finger down my throat.... I wiped off the toilet and began rinsing my beet red face when I was startled by a hard knock on the door. "Cherry, what's going on?" My father's voice was stern....

God, what's wrong with me? Why can't I control myself? If I just hadn't have tasted that turkey, then I wouldn't have gorged and had to throw up and lie to Daddy. But, I had to eat something. I hadn't eaten all day! I looked at my swollen eyes as tears streaked down my hallow cheeks. I leaned against the door and slid down slowly as my whining turned to uncontrollable sobbing. God, take me, please! I can't handle this anymore! I don't want to live like this forever, Take me, please! The idea of facing another day terrified me. The only thing that had kept me going this far was a faint, flickering, inner spark of hope — hope that somehow, someday, there would be the "way out" I so desperately needed. And, that spark was fading fast. I had no idea I was slowly committing suicide.[6]

Eating disorders affect young people as well as adults. Anorexia nervosa is a self-induced starvation resulting in extreme weight loss and characterized by an intense fear of gaining weight. One in every one hundred women suffers from it. Some anorexics are also bulimic in their behavior. Bulimia is a pattern of bingeing (eating large amounts of food) followed by self-induced vomiting or laxative abuse with or without weight loss. When people eat large amounts of food to satisfy emotional hungers (hungers of which they may or may not be aware) compulsive overeating becomes the pattern. The compulsive overeater may be a few pounds or a few hundred pounds overweight. Studies show that an overweight adolescent is more likely to become an overweight adult. Overweight adults can have physical as well as emotional problems related to their eating disorder.

Although eating disorders typically affect young females between the ages of twelve and eighteen, a small percentage of young boys suffer from them, too. The pattern developed at a young age can continue into adulthood. An eating disorder can become a secret nightmare from which each victim and family desires desperately to escape.

## 1 Know the Causes

What causes eating disorders? According to Dr. Paul Meier of the Minirth-Meier Clinic, the causes of eating disorders are like the different segments of a multi-colored beach ball. There are many different causes. People need to see all sides of the beach ball in order to answer this question accurately. Just as there is not one single cure for an eating disorder, there is also not one single cause.

There is much debate surrounding the causes of eating disorders — especially anorexia and bulimia. Some physicians view anorexia as a symptom of a deeper disease while others see it as a separate one. Even though these two theories approach anorexia differently, the most important fact is that they both share the desire of bringing healing to the anorexic.

As a health educator, I see nothing wrong with accepting the idea that an individual may have a biological predisposition to an eating disorder. Besides possibly having a biological predisposition to the disease, we should also be aware of:

## *Physical factors:*

- Possible link between anorexia and severe zinc deficiency[7]

## *Social factors:*

- Pressure from society and peers to be thin

- Feelings of unacceptance

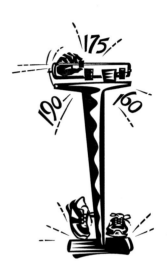

## *Personal factors:*

- Family dynamics: divorce, separation, abuse, death of family member, emotionally absent parent(s), frequent conflict between daughter and mother

- Stress: academic, athletic, competition of any sort

- Tendency to be a perfectionist

- Using food as a sedative, form of comfort, or as an attempt to fill one's empty "love tank"

- Desire to take personal control over something in life when other areas are out of control

- Excessive teasing from family members or peers concerning weight

## *Eating Disorders and the Addiction Cycle*

One of the main contributing factors to teens' eating disorders is unmet emotional needs. In an attempt to fulfill their unmet emotional needs, especially their need for love, some teens choose to turn to food or thinness (body image) as their solution.

This can set in motion a cycle of obsession/compulsion/addiction from which it can be very difficult for teens to escape.

The addiction cycle is comprised of seven downward steps. Each step leads to the next when teens' inner needs are not met. The steps are:

1. Teens' hunger for love is not satisfied.

2. Teens feel emotional pain, low self-esteem.

3. Teens choose food as an anesthetic for their pain.

4. Teens begin to experience the addictive consequences of their anesthetic.

5. Teens feel guilty and/or shameful for their unhealthy behavior.

6. Teens feel a self-hatred for continuing in their unhealthy behavior.

7. Teens' hunger for love remains unsatisfied.

When teenagers' hunger for love is not met, they experience some form of emotional pain, usually resulting in a feeling of low self-esteem. If they are unwilling or unable to allow God to fill their needs for love and worth, they begin to use food or thinness as an anesthetic to dull their inner emotional pain. The more they continue to try to use food or thinness to satisfy their emotional needs without God, the more that food or thinness become a driving obsession, which then turns into a true addiction. Since neither food nor thinness can satisfy teens' needs for love and worth, they begin to experience the consequences of their compulsive behavior (e.g., obesity, anorexia, bulimia). The teens that grow up in Christian homes know instinctively that their choices are unhealthy. They feel a legitimate guilt for their behavior because they sense that they are not going in the direction that their loving heavenly Father would want them to go. They then begin to feel a sense of guilt for their behavior. If they can acknowledge their need and sense a ray of hope, they can be motivated to turn to God's grace to change them by allowing Him to meet their deep needs for love and worth.

Many teenagers with eating disorders, however, don't turn to God to meet their deepest desires. If they don't turn toward God to fulfill their emotional needs; but instead continue to listen to the unhealthy messages communicated to them from media, peers, and even possibly their own parents; and, if they do not receive some professional help; they may judge themselves as worthless persons — drowning themselves in shame. Their unmanageable addiction only adds to their inner self-rejection and feelings of shame. If they do not find answers at this stage of the addiction cycle, then self-hatred sets in. If left unresolved, self-hatred only continues the addiction cycle. When teens use food or thinness to try to make themselves not feel self-hatred, they only find again that food or thinness do not satisfy; thus the cycle goes on and on. [8]

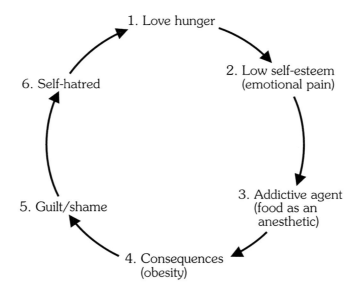

1. Love hunger

2. Low self-esteem
(emotional pain)

3. Addictive agent
(food as an
anesthetic)

4. Consequences
(obesity)

5. Guilt/shame

6. Self-hatred

There is a lot of denial involved in eating disorders because they are forms of addiction. Both anorexics and bulimics deny the reality of their physical bodies.

> "Eating-disordered persons will see themselves as heavier or lighter than they are — and that is a part of their denial, a key aspect of addiction. Any addiction destroys the person's ability to see objectively."[9]

I can say from personal observation, that it is very easy for parents and family members also to be in denial about the presence of eating disorders in the lives of those who are close to them. My family ignored the deeper emotional issues underlying the anorexia of my older sister, Ann. Instead of seeking professional help for her, my family placed its energies on getting her to eat more food. Because of our ignorance of eating disorders, all of us thought that Ann was just on a very strict diet.

If you have a child who might have an eating disorder, ignoring the situation will not make it go away. The hardest step may be to let the truth come out. When the truth is revealed, the process of healing can begin.

Because of their increasing interest in social interaction and eventual dating, courtship, and marriage, it is not unusual for teens — as well as adults — to want to diet and lose weight. The key is noticing unhealthy eating patterns. Answer the following questions to the best of your knowledge concerning your teen. If you have a concern about her eating habits at school, call one of your teen's teachers to discuss it.

## 2 Observe Your Teen

The following questions will help you to see whether or not your teen shows any signs of an eating disorder.

### *Anorexia nervosa:*

- Has your teen lost a significant amount of weight recently?
  Yes / No / I don't know

- Does your teen think that she is too heavy or too thin? Yes / No / I don't know

- Does your teen seem to have an obsession with exercise (never seems to miss a day of exercise; arranges schedule around physical workouts; insists on one or two workouts a day; wants to exercise even when sick)?
  Yes / No / I don't know

- Does your teen seem generally healthy to you? Yes / No / I don't know

- Does your child seem abnormally tired or weak much of the time?
  Yes / No / I don't know

- Does your teen seem extremely picky about the food she eats (always makes her own dinner; eats very small portions; consistently leaves food on her plate)? Yes / No / I don't know

- Has your daughter experienced amenorrhea (absence of monthly menstruation)? Yes / No / I don't know

    If so, how much of the time: 10%, 20%, 30%, or more?

## *Bulimia*

- Does your teen complain about ridicule at school concerning her weight?
  Yes / No / I don't know

- Does your teen eat in private much of the time? Yes / No / I don't know

- Does your teen eat mainly to satisfy an emotional need, e.g., depression, anger, or disappointment? Yes / No / I don't know

- Does your child induce vomiting after meals? (One clue would be if she spent a lot of extra time in the bathroom claiming that she was sick.)
  Yes / No / I don't know

- Does your teen use laxatives to lose weight? (Have you noticed any laxatives in the bathroom)? Yes / No / I don't know

- Has your daughter experienced amenorrhea (absence of monthly menstruation)? Yes / No / I don't know

- Does your teen eat large amounts of food? Yes / No / I don't know

- Have you noticed food hidden in your teen's room, closet, or other locations where she might eat unnoticed? Yes / No / I don't know

## *Overeating*

- Is your teen significantly overweight? Yes / No / I don't know

- Does your teen complain about ridicule at school concerning his weight?
  Yes / No / I don't know

- Have you noticed food hidden in your teen's room, closet, or other locations where he might eat unnoticed? Yes / No / I don't know

- Does your teen regularly eat while he is watching TV or movies? If so, what kind of food does he eat, and in what quantity?
Yes / No / I don't know

- Does your child eat large amounts of food?
Yes / No / I don't know

- Does your child eat to satisfy unmet emotional needs? For instance, does he/she eat a lot more food when depressed, angry, or disappointed?
Yes / No / I don't know

- Does your child openly talk about his weight problem and sincerely want to change? Yes / No / I don't know

> "Teenagers equate failure with weakness, casting stones at themselves when overweight leaves too slowly or stays. They cement self-worth to society's dictum to be thin; at all costs be thin. Believing looks and worth are one and the same, they put shape in charge of self-esteem... Success of a program seeks observable changes: buy fewer rich foods; visit the bakery less often; play basketball, football, volleyball more often; watch TV less; avoid rigid diets to avoid self-defeating hunger. Search not for flaws in character, but for changes of behavior."[10]

If you find that your teen shows signs of compulsive overeating after answering the previous questions on this subject, you can choose one of the following three options presented by Michael LeBow, Ph.D., in his book, *Overweight Teenagers*.[11] Depending upon your personal situation, choose the option that best suits your teen's needs:

1. **Wait-and-see.** If you feel your teen has a problem, but it hasn't become acute, then you may choose to wait-and-see how he matures. Your teen may also exhibit a very good self-image despite being overweight. This healthy attitude will be significant in choosing which option best fits your teen.

2. **Promote small changes.** If you feel your teen has a problem, but it doesn't seem to be a serious health risk, you may want to encourage small changes. Talk to your teen about his feelings toward school, friends, and family. Let him know you care and love him just the way he is. Tell your teen you want to make some nutritional changes for the whole family. Don't single your child out. Also, try to interest your teen in family exercises and activities.

3. **Promote large changes.** If you feel your teen is at risk and is open to more drastic changes, then you may want to promote large changes. Have your teen be an active participant in choosing the program. If you choose this option, the family and parents together with the teen become actively involved in the process. The following are a few ideas to get teens involved in their own recovery.

- Ask your teen to help design and/or finance a program for a change of eating habits.

- Get your teen involved in stocking nutritious, low-fat foods that make the program run smoothly.

- Have everyone create menus together.

- Decide exercise programs with each other.

- Have everyone see a physician regularly.

- Set small, attainable goals which build confidence and competency.

- Read a book on recovery together.

## 3 Talk with Your Teen

If your child has an eating disorder at any stage, it is essential that she admits that she has a problem and is willing to receive help. Use the following questions to engage your teen in conversation about what might be happening deep inside of her. Your goal is to try to get her to admit that she might be using food or thinness as a way of meeting her need for love and self-worth; needs that only God can satisfy. After reading all of the following questions, choose which ones would be the most effective ways for you to use to begin a casual conversation with your teen.

Remember that your purpose is to get your teen to open up — not shut down as a result of you dominating the conversation.

- *"Do you honestly feel loved by those close to you in your life? If not, who do you feel really doesn't love you? What do they do or say to you that makes you feel unloved?"*

- *"Do you honestly feel accepted by those close to you in your life? If not, who do you feel really doesn't accept you? What do they do or say to you that makes you feel unaccepted?"*

- *"How do you really feel about yourself? Do you feel good about yourself or do you feel that you have to please others, get high grades, be a star on the basketball team, have certain guys or girls like you, or get other's approval before you can feel good about yourself?"*

- *"Do you think that someone could actually so dislike themselves inside, that they start to do self-destructive activities? If so, what kinds of self-destructive behaviors have you seen other people do? Why do you think that they do them?"*

- *"Do you like the way that God has made you? If you were standing in front of a mirror, and had the power to change anything that you wanted, would you change anything? If so, what? Why?"*

- *"Jesus said to love our neighbor as we love ourselves. Do you think that people need to love themselves before they can love others? Do you think that it is right, wrong, or in-between to love yourself? Do you love yourself? Is there any part of you that you could say that you strongly dislike?"*

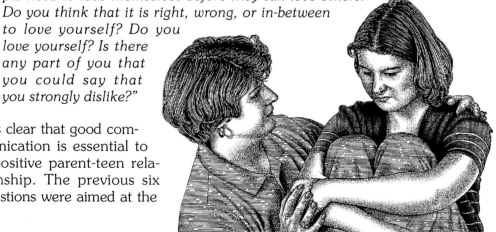

It is clear that good communication is essential to a positive parent-teen relationship. The previous six questions were aimed at the possible deeper causes of eating disorders. They were indirect questions. If you wanted to approach the subject more directly with your teen, you could simply turn to some of the questions in an earlier part of this section and re-word them. Remember, however, that a teen that shows signs of a serious eating disorder has most likely begun to withdraw. As a result of what the teen is experiencing, communication may be strained if not non-existent.

Another factor is that an individual suffering from an eating disorder has begun a cycle of denial/deception. Lying about their eating habits becomes a pattern of survival. Therefore, the approach in this section concentrates on observing your teen's behavior and emotions. Make notes of your observations. Get the opinion of significant others in your child's life. Discuss the situation with your spouse, a teacher, youth pastor, or close adult. Above all, show your teen unconditional love and acceptance.

#  Take Action

When making observations concerning your teen, it's possible to feel overwhelmed with the seriousness of the issues. Worry can set in, and we can begin to feel helpless. The goal of *The Parent Connection* is not only to assist you in seeing the problem, but also to enable you to know what to do about it. These Action Steps will help you to get a handle on the pertinent information that will show you how to proceed.

After making careful observations, try to place your teen in one of the following categories:

❏ **Category 1:** Your teen shows no signs of having an eating disorder. (If so, you may stop here and move on to another teen issue in *The Parent Connection*.)

❏ **Category 2:** Your teen shows potential signs of having an eating disorder.

A teen that shows potential signs will be dealing with low self-esteem, equating looks and/or thinness with value, a self-hatred cycle, control issues, and even possibly hiding and deceiving. Teens' deceitfulness will involve lying concerning what they have or have not eaten. If your teen shows any potential signs of an eating disorder, here are some professional suggestions as to what to do and what not to do:

Do:

- Fill his "love tank" with positive things concerning his inner person.

- Give physical encouragement to your teen, a touch or hug.

- Help your teen face her problems. Let her know you are interested and involved. Nothing is too insignificant.

- Plan to introduce healthy meals for the benefit of the whole family.

- Gain the counsel of someone trained in the area of eating disorders.

- Read a good book to help you better understand your teen.

- Educate the rest of the family so they are more sensitive to the situation.

- Initiate talk about the activities, friends, places, stores, sports, books, games, videos, etc. that interest your teen to build a bridge of positive 7communication.

- Recognize there's a problem.

- Continue to take note of your teen's behavior and emotional changes, whether positive or negative.

Don't:

- Discuss the way he looks or how much he weighs (unless he has already admitted that he has a problem and has expressed a desire to change).

- Mention the fact that you have noticed that he has put on a few pounds. (This goes for the anorexic, bulimic, and overeater).

- Try to force her to eat.

- Try consciously to fix her favorite foods in an attempt to motivate her to eat more food.

- Threaten your teen with rewards and punishments related to her eating habits. (Do this only if your teen is on a program that she has agreed to do.)

- Try to analyze or counsel her without professional input.

- Tell her that "everyone is worried about her" and have noticed her changing.

- Treat your teen differently than the rest of your children.

- Preach at her about how badly she is treating the "temple of the Holy Spirit."

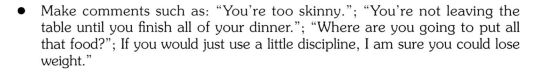

- Ignore the situation by thinking that it's just a "phase" and will go away.

- Make comments such as: "You're too skinny."; "You're not leaving the table until you finish all of your dinner."; "Where are you going to put all that food?"; If you would just use a little discipline, I am sure you could lose weight."

❏ **Category 3:** Your teen shows signs of having an advanced case of an eating disorder. If you notice that your teen shows signs of having an advanced case of an eating disorder, communication may be very difficult. As you recognize the severity of the situation, focus on building a bridge of awareness with your teen and begin to seek professional guidance. Remember that your teen has a distorted view of her body and her source of self-worth. She is unable to see reality objectively. Your teen needs your help. Professional medical attention and counseling is vital at this stage.

Do:

- Show total, unconditional love and acceptance to your teen.

- Seek professional help without delay.

- Tell your teen that the reason that you're going to seek professional help for her is because you really love her.

- Communicate to your teen how much God unconditionally loves and cares for her.

- Encourage your teen with the fact that God will actively give grace as she asks Him for it.

- Take the situation seriously without denying any aspect of it.

- Ask everyone in your immediate family to stop all teasing and sarcasm toward your teen.

Don't:

- Panic!

- Ask her, "How could you do this to us?"

- Ask her, "How could you do this to yourself?"

- Yell or nag at her about her eating habits.

❏ After this section, do you feel that your teen has an eating disorder? If so, what name would you give it?
  - Anorexia?
  - Bulimia?
  - Combination of Anorexia and Bulimia?
  - Overeating?

❏ List below the three most important "do's" that your family needs to work on:

_____

_____

_____

❏ List below the three most important "do not's" that your family needs to work on:

_____

_____

_____

❏ After going through this section, do you feel that you need to call a family meeting without the teen who is suffering from this eating disorder? If so:

- Date and location of meeting planned:_____

  _____

- Things you need to discuss at this family meeting:

  _____

  _____

  _____

❏ Do you want to read some books on eating disorders? If so, list them here:

  _____

  _____

❏ Do you want to contact an organization or professional to help? If so, list them here:

  _____

  _____

## *5* Pause to Reflect

After you finish the appropriate Action Steps, complete this evaluation to see how the chapter worked for you.

- How well did you "connect" with your teen on this issue?

  Not very well          Fairly well          Very well

- What did you learn about your teen that you did not know before this section?




- What did you learn about your family as a result of this connection?




- What did you learn about yourself as a result of this material?

- How successful were the Action Steps in your situation?

  Not successful          Somewhat successful          Very successful

- Record any further insights, questions, or comments concerning this section and your teen below:

## Further Resources

### *Associations:*

American Anorexia/Bulimia Association
293 Central Park West Suite 1R
New York, NY. 10024
(212) 501–8351

ANRED
Anorexia Nervosa and Related Eating Disorders
P.O. Box 5102
Eugene, OR. 97405
(503) 344–1144

Institute for the Study of Anorexia and Bulimia
1 West 91st Street
New York, NY 10024
(212) 595–3449

National Eating Disorders Organization
445 E. Granville Road
Worthington, OH. 43085–3195
(614) 436–1112

## Books:

*Walking the Thin Line, Anorexia and Bulimia, the Battle Can Be Won*, Pam Vredevelt. (Multnomah Press, 1985).

*The Thin Disguise*, Pam Vredevelt, et. al., (Thomas Nelson, 1992).

*Hope, Help & Healing For Eating Disorders, A New Approach To Treating Anorexia, Bulimia and Overeating*, Gregory L. Jantz PhD. (Harold Shaw Publishers, 1995).

*The Monster Within, Overcoming Bulimia*, Cynthia Joe Rowland, (Baker Book House, 1984).

*Starving for Attention*, Cherry Boone O'Neill, (Dell Publishing, New York, 1982).

*Love Hunger: Recovery from Food Addiction*, Frank Minirth, et. al., (Thomas Nelson, Nashville, 1990).

*Overweight Teenagers Don't Bear the Burden Alone*, Michael D. LeBow, (Plenum Press: Insight Books, New York, 1995).

# CHAPTER THREE

# Over-Exercising

*Many teens find it difficult to work even seemingly normal diets because, impatient for results, they fall victim to the "more is better" fallacy... Fueling this fallacy is the hurry-up attitude of "I want change, and I want it fast." Impatience forecasts trouble....[12]*

The desire for instant results is not the only factor influencing teens' decisions. Drs. Minirth and Meier put it this way: "Adults as well as teens are constantly being bombarded by cultural pressures to 'eat, eat, eat' or 'get slim, slim, slim!' Never before in history have so much time, money, and energy gone into urging people to eat and yet at the same time demanding that they be slim. Psychiatrists call these push/pull messages, double-bind messages, paradox messages, or, best of all, crazy-making messages."[13]

It's easy to see how teenagers can over-eat or under-eat in response to these crazy-making bombardments. In a similar way, the issue of exercising also involves push/pull messages for teens. On the over-exercise side, the promotion of hundreds of exercise videos, the home exercise equipment craze in department stores and on cable TV, and the push for athletic club memberships all communicate to teens the message: "Exercise more!"

On the under-exercise side, sports medicine is clearly trying to down scale the hard core exerciser with its promotion of the adequacy of three 20-minute workouts per week, its soft emphasis involving "use the stairs instead of the elevator," and its publishing articles of how certain exercises, when incorrectly executed, can actually damage the body. Moreover, when busy or lazy teens constantly hear the messages of the over-exercisers, their internal self-talk understandably promotes their shying away from exercise. For their own emotional survival, they tell themselves,

"Academics are more important;" "I have no time;" "Walking home from school and walking around the mall is enough;" or, "It's too difficult to begin an exercise program, since I'll probably end up quitting anyway." When teens receive so many contradictory messages, they feel pressure to have to choose who they are going to believe and how much exercise they are going to fit into their lives.

# 1 Know the Causes

As parents, we must remember that there's a fine line between teens who exercise to maintain fitness and teens who are obsessed with fitness. When teens' "workouts" become the center of their daily schedule, an imbalance can occur, resulting in an obsession. To prevent such an imbalance in your own teen's life, begin to develop answers to the following questions: When does exercise become "over-exercise?" When exactly can a teen know that he is under-exercising? How can a teenager exercise too much? Isn't over-exercising better than not exercising at all?

When it comes to answering these questions for your teen, the most important point to keep in mind is not so much how many times per week your teen is exercising, but why he is exercising and how exercising is affecting the other areas of his life. If your teen tends to be an over-exerciser, he's probably dealing with much more than only the desire to be fit. Consider the various causes for over-exercising. An individual who over-exercises may:

- Be responding to the media messages from society to be fit.

- Desire subconsciously to control some area in his life.

- Use exercise as an escape from an emotional hurt.

- Use exercise as an antidepressant.

- Use exercise to please others and self.

- Use exercise to avoid facing his problems, responsibilities, or relationships.

- Use exercise to have a feeling of "belonging."

- Use exercise to mask other problems he's having.

- Use exercise to gain a sense of personal accomplishment or competency.

- Use exercise as a way to satisfy an inner drive to compete and win.

- Use exercise in response to low self-esteem.

As you probably noticed, not all of the causes of over-exercising are bad in themselves. As a matter of fact, exercise can be a good, legitimate outlet for many of the stresses teens and adults face. Problems occur when a teen's life begins to revolve around exercise. The following are some danger signs that indicate that exercise has probably become too important in a teen's life.

- When a teen feels that his next workout must be much more intense and difficult than usual in an effort to make up for the workout he may have missed the time before.

- When a teen always schedules his day around his workout time.

- When a teen frequently damages or neglects his other responsibilities, homework, family, friends, and personal health for the sake of maintaining his exercise routine.

## A Note about STEROIDS AND ERGOGENIC AIDS:

An ergogenic aid is something that improves physical work performance. Anything from a strict diet to anabolic steroids has been used to help athletes feel they have an edge over the competition. Anabolic steroids are synthetic forms of the male hormone testosterone. Testosterone is the hormone responsible for the development of secondary sex characteristics in males. The negative side effects of steroid usage include: stunted growth, liver damage, strokes, heart disease, and possible infertility. In women, steroid use may result in a disruption of the menstrual cycle and may lead to an increase in masculine physical features. If you feel your son or daughter may be involved in the use of steroids, find out the facts, and then take your teen to see a physician who can explain the negative consequences of steroid use.

## 2 Observe Your Teen

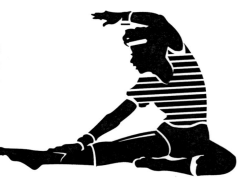

It's very healthy for teens to exercise. There [is nothing?]
wrong with them enjoying the discipline and [that?]
exercise demands. As you make the following [observations?]
concerning your teen, try to look beyond the [fact that he?]
enjoys exercising. Do you see any deeper unm[et emo]tional needs in him that may be causing him
to use exercising as a way of filling voids that
only God can fill?

- How often does your teen workout?
  Once a day / Twice a day / Three or more times a day

- Does your teen complain when he cannot have a workout?
  Yes / No / I don't know

- If your teen is involved in sports, does he/she still workout the same day as team practice? Yes / No / I don't know

- Does your teen exercise even more when angry, depressed, or emotionally hurt? Yes / No / I don't know

- Does your teen insist on exercising even when sick?
  Yes / No / I don't know

- Does your teen seem inflexible when it comes to his workout times?
  Yes / No / I don't know

- Does your teen keep detailed records, charts, or journals all centered around workout goals? Yes / No / I don't know

- Does your teen belong to an athletic club or gym?
  Yes / No / I don't know

- If your teen belongs to an athletic club, does he spend more time there than you feel is appropriate? Yes / No / I don't know

- Does your teen spend a lot of his money on athletic equipment, workout magazines, designer clothes, sport shoes, and/or accessories?
  Yes / No / I don't know

- Does your teen seem to be obsessed with weightlifting and his physique?
  Yes / No / I don't know

- Does your teen seem isolated from your family because he's so consumed with his fitness program? Yes / No / I don't know

- Have you seen a marked increase in your teen's muscular development?
  Yes / No / I don't know

- Are you concerned that your teen may be taking steroids?
  Yes / No / I don't know

- Does your teen often have injuries related to sports/exercise?
  Yes / No / I don't know

- Do any other members in your family exhibit any similar obsession?
  Yes / No / I don't know

## *3* Talk with Your Teen

If, after answering the preceding questions, you feel that your teen is obsessed with exercise and fitness, you may want to use the following Conversation Starters to see if there is a deeper reason for this imbalance. After reading all of the following questions, choose which ones would be the most effective ways for you to use to begin a casual conversation with your teen. Remember that your purpose is to get your teen to open up — not shut down as a result of you dominating the conversation.

- *"How does it make you feel when you workout?"*

- *"When you miss your workout how does it make you feel?"*

- *"I've noticed that you take your workouts very seriously. I'm proud of your discipline and hard work. How do you feel about your accomplishment?"*

- *"What kind of messages about yourself are you receiving from your peers? What kind of messages about yourself are you receiving from the adults in your life?"*

- *"Is it difficult for you to engage in recreational activities without feeling that they need to be an intense workout?"*

- *"If you could do any activity just for fun, what would you choose and why?"*

- *"If you could be any sports figure, living or dead, who would you be and why?"*

- *"If you had an unlimited amount of time and money, what would you do with your life? Where would you go?"*

- *"How would you feel if you were suddenly unable to exercise due to a serious injury? What would you do instead of exercise?"*

- *"Do you feel satisfied with the friendships you have? Who would you say is your best friend? Why is he/she such a good friend?"*

- *"Do you know any one who uses steroids to enhance his appearance or performance? What do you think of using steroids?"*

- *"When you lose a game, how do you feel (angry, disappointed, like a failure)?"*

- *"Is it difficult for you to play any game without always feeling intensely competitive?"*

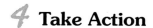

## 🍀 Take Action

After using the Conversation Starters with your teen in an attempt to "connect" with him/her using open communication, you may feel you are not making any progress. It's helpful to remember that teens don't always know "why" they do things. Neither do they always know exactly how they feel about something. They may simply say to you, "I like exercise because it makes me feel good." If you have discovered that your teen does have an obsession with exercise/fitness, consider the following Action Steps to help bring constructive change into your teen's life.

## ❏ Interview with the Coach:

Talk to your teen's coach or school counselor about his fitness habits at school. It's important to keep in mind that a coach has a tendency to think positively about an athlete who goes beyond the call of duty, putting extra hours into practicing or working out. For this reason, your teen's coach may not share your same concerns.

Nevertheless, you can ask the coach the following questions:

- Does my son work out before or after practice?
- Does my son seem overly intense concerning this sport?
- Does my daughter isolate herself from her teammates?
- Does my daughter seem to have unrealistic expectations of herself?
- What observations do you have concerning my son/daughter?

## ❏ Self-Opinion Letter:

Each person (both parent and teen) take a clean sheet of paper and complete this sentence as fully as you can: "I don't like myself because…" An honest assessment of the answer will be helpful in two ways. It may bring up valid areas where self-improvement is needed, but more importantly, it will show areas of unnecessary self-blame.

On another sheet of paper, write a letter of introduction for yourself, commending yourself to a new person you will be meeting. Generously list all of your positive qualities. In this exercise, give yourself full permission to lay aside all self-criticism. If possible, read aloud this list of attributes to each other. This sharing may seem awkward, but it is a powerful means of positively reinforcing yourself and your teen. [14]

❏ Are you or your spouse going to talk to some significant people concerning your teen's obsession with exercise? If so, please list their names below:

- _____
- _____
- _____

# *5* **Pause to Reflect**

After you finish the appropriate Action Steps, complete this evaluation to see how the chapter worked for you.

- How well did you "connect" with your teen in this section?

  Not very well          Fairly well          Very well

- What did you learn about your teen that you did not know before this connection?



- What did you learn about your family as a result of this section?



- What did you learn about yourself as a result of this material?



- How successful were the Action Steps for your situation?

  Not successful          Somewhat successful          Very successful

- Record any further insights, questions, or comments concerning this section and your teen here:

# Under-Exercising

*Judging from the numbers of teenagers who diet, you must agree that many, if not most teens, would rather eat less than move more; would rather fast than walk a few extra miles or play a few extra hours of sports... for the sake of your body, your emotions, [and] your outlook, live the active life. Because overweight and inactivity often share the same body...* [15]

Parents who eat right, exercise regularly, and are motivated to maintain good health disciplines, tend to look at overweight teens and wonder, "Why can't they just discipline themselves more?!" Healthy and slender parents who have never had a weight problem, have difficulty empathizing with the overweight teenager because they have never experienced being: laughed at because of how they looked in a swimsuit, called "fatso" or "thunder thighs," ignored socially, picked last for a team, or, the object of cruel jokes. Conversely, those parents who have experienced the pain of being overweight — in a society where fit equates with "strong" and fat equates with "weak"— can understand why even some teens have such low activity levels.

## 1 Know the Causes

Michael D. LeBow explains a few of the barriers that keep teens from becoming active in his book, *Overweight Teenagers: Don't Bear the Burden Alone.* They are:

- **Fear of Embarrassment:** Overweight teens fear the ridicule of those who may watch them and laugh at their efforts or movements. They would rather sit in front of a nonjudgmental TV than experience the pain associated with activity.

- **Overdoing:** When feeling highly motivated, overweight teens might make an effort to exercise. In a gallant effort to lose weight quickly, however, they might workout too hard. Consequently, they discover that they were unable to maintain such high standards. Their body was not ready for such a shock. Failure sets in. By attempting too much too soon, they get discouraged and quit.

- **Boredom:** "I hate exercise" is a common complaint from teens who get bored with anything having to do with activity. Feeling incompetent might be the true cause behind the boredom.

- **Schedule Disruption:** Oftentimes, motivated teenagers make specific plans for their day. They might think, "I will get up at 6:30AM and walk 30 minutes before school;" then an unplanned circumstance disrupts their schedule. If this happens too many times, a loss of motivation results. To avoid such discouragement, support your teen's exercise plans.

## 2 Observe Your Teen

Unless teens are involved in an organized athletic activity, it's unlikely that they will maintain a consistent exercise program on their own. Note the following observations of your teen when determining the extent of their sedentary lifestyle:

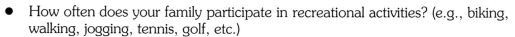

- How much TV does your teen watch each day?

  1 hour or less     2–3 hours     4 hours or more

- How overweight is your teen?

  5–10 pounds     10–20 pounds     20 pounds or more

- How often does your family participate in recreational activities? (e.g., biking, walking, jogging, tennis, golf, etc.)

  Less than once a week          2–3 times a week          4 times a week or more

- What is your teen's attitude toward activity and movement?

  Enjoys any activity     Enjoys noncompetitive activity     Sedentary; dislikes activity and movement

- What is your family's general attitude toward exercise and activity?

  Enjoys any activity     Enjoys noncompetitive activity     Sedentary; dislikes activity and movement

- Does your teen engage in negative self-talk?  Yes / No / I don't know

- If yes, how intensely?
  Somewhat negative      Very negative      Always negative

## 3 Talk with Your Teen

After honestly answering the previous observations of your teen and family, you may want to use the following Conversation Starters to encourage your teen to live a more active life. After reading all of the following questions, choose which ones would be the most effective ways for you to use to begin a casual conversation with your teen. Remember that your purpose is to get your teen to open up — not shut down as a result of you dominating the conversation.

- *"Do you enjoy sports?"*

- *"What sports do you enjoy?"*

- *"Who usually plays the sport(s) with you?"*

- *"How do you feel about our family walks?" "Would you like to start walking with the family?"*

- *"Do others tease you about your weight?" "In what ways?" "How often?" "What sorts of things do they say?"*

- *"Do you think it's healthier to be overweight or underweight?"*

- *"What role do you think exercise has in good health?"*

- *"If you could participate in any Olympic event what would it be?"*

- *"How do you feel about setting goals for exercise?"*

- *"Do you enjoy Physical Education class at school?"*

- *"What motivates you to do things that you normally don't like to do?"*

# 4 Take Action

After using the previous Conversation Starters with your teen, do you feel that he has an unhealthy view of exercise? If so, what seems to be the main barrier to him exercising more? (If necessary, review the list of barriers in the Causes section.) When trying to encourage your teen to become more active, it's important to help him think positively about the program or activity that is planned. It's also beneficial for the whole family to get involved. Exercise is good for everyone, not only those who are overweight. Consider the following Action Steps to help implement more activity into your teen's life.

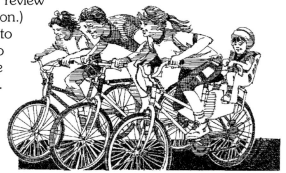

❑ **Talk to your teen's Physical Education teacher.** What activities is your teen good at during class? What is your teen's attitude during class? What suggestions do they have to motivate your teen?

❑ **Keep an exercise journal.** Your teen can use the same journal for both food and exercise.

❑ **Set some family exercise goals.** For example, bike riding on weekends and/or a family walk three times a week.

❑ **Limit time spent watching TV**, movies and/or playing video games.

❑ **Make some reading commitments.** For example, I'm going to read the following book(s) on exercise:

_____

_____

_____

_____

_____

_____

# *5* **Pause to Reflect**

After you finish the appropriate Action Steps, complete this evaluation to see how the chapter worked for you.

- How well did you "connect" with your teen in this section?

  Not very well          Fairly well          Very well

- What have you learned about your teen that you did not know before?

- What did you discover about your family as a result of this material?

- What did this connection teach you about yourself?

- How successful were the Action Steps for your situation?

  Not successful          Somewhat successful          Very successful

- Record any further insights, questions, or comments concerning under-exercising and your teen below:

## Further Resources

*Love Hunger: Recovery from Food Addiction*, Dr. Frank Minirth, et. al. (Thomas Nelson Publishers, 1990).

*Thoroughly Fit, How To Make Lifestyle Changes In 90 Days: Physical, Spiritual, Emotional, Mental*, Becky Tirabassi and Candice Copeland Brooks, (Zondervan, 1993).

*Greater Health God's Way*, Stormie Omartian, (Harvest House, 1996).

*Overweight Teenagers: Don't Bear The Burden Alone*, Michael D. LeBow, (Plenum Press, 1995).

# Infectious Diseases

*After God let the Israelites out of Egypt, He promised His people that if they would obey His statutes, He would put "none of these diseases" upon them. Was this a trustworthy promise? Could submitting to a code of "restrictive" rules lead to freedom from sicknesses? Could this promise remain pertinent even in the twentieth century? Yes! Obedience to biblical precepts is still the most effective way to prevent many of the afflictions of mankind.[16]*

Many people think that sickness is "just a part of life." Aches, pains, constant fatigue, frequent battle with colds, and the general feeling of unhealthiness has kept the medical community in high demand. Too many of us want a quick fix for symptoms that may have developed over a period of many years. Generally speaking, treatment has taken precedence over prevention. Prevention takes discipline and knowledge. If a person wants to avoid illness and its symptoms, then prevention is the best medicine. As the old adage says, "An ounce of prevention is worth a pound of cure." Prevention addresses a teen's lifestyle choices as well as his/her thoughts and attitudes. Preventative medicine, however, runs contrary to a promiscuous and indulgent society. It can, however, be successfully implemented into an entire family's lifestyle.

## *1* Know the Causes

All diseases that are caused by the spread of germ (or pathogen) microorganisms are called infectious. They are known as "communicable" diseases because they can be passed on from one person to another. Pathogens include: bacteria, viruses, fungi, and tiny animals.

### The Process of Infection

Pathogen ➡ Host ➡ Spreading ➡ New Host

The infectious disease process includes four factors: the pathogen itself, the source of the pathogen, the spread of the pathogen, and the new host. The germ must be destroyed during the infectious disease process or the sickness will continue to spread. Germs use two main ways to escape from their existing host. One escape is through the respiratory tract by way of sneezing or coughing. When a person sneezes or coughs, the germs travel through the air by way of tiny droplets. The tiny droplets provide the germs a warm and moist environment in which they normally thrive. Their other exit is through the intestinal tract by way of feces.

Germs are spread through direct contact with an:
- infected person,
- infected animal (e.g., bites), or
- infected object (through being touched by an infected person).

Disease development requires an incubation period for the germ. The incubation period begins the moment people become infected with a microorganism to the time when they actually experience the symptoms of the intruder. The incubation period is the most infectious time of the disease. It's called the contagious period. The contagious period is often difficult to pinpoint because it's usually during the very early stages of the sickness. Infected individuals may not even realize that they are spreading the disease. The symptoms that people feel actually allow them to recognize the presence and type of the disease.

Physicians prescribe antibiotics to children who suffer from bacterial infections. Antibiotics, however, are not always necessary. Sometimes the body can fight off a bacterial infection if its immune system is strong and healthy. Without antibiotics, however, the healing process is slower. Natural recuperation also takes more discipline in the areas of healthy eating and getting sufficient rest.

When individuals suffer from a cold, they are suffering from a virus and not a bacteria. Viruses are responsible for more infections than any other pathogen. While bacteria produce toxins in the body, viruses attack individual cells. The virus chooses the tissue it wants to damage and then invades the cells of the tissue. For example, polio viruses invade the cells of the nervous system; cold sore viruses invade the cells of the skin; and flu viruses attack the cells of the respiratory system. Viruses are also responsible for mumps, measles, chicken pox, smallpox, rabies, AIDS, and most cases of hepatitis.

# 2 Observe Your Teen

It's my observation that teens usually have more going on in their minds than what they let you know. Concerning illness, I've found that adolescents can be divided into three general categories. Note which of the following categories best describes your teen:

**The Silent Sufferer:** This teenager does not tell you how he really feels because:

- he fears that he may have a serious disease; and/or
- he fears that you will make him miss desirable activities; and/or
- he does not want to seem weak or "wimpy"; and/or
- he does not want to go to the doctor.

**The Hypochondriac:** This teenager constantly complains about every symptom she has because:

- she fears that he may have a serious disease; and/or
- she's hungry for attention; and/or
- she heard about a person who had the same symptoms and was very sick; and/or
- she's using illness as an escape from responsibility.

**The Strong One:** This teenager has a good attitude when sick because:

- he has a good sense of security about self and home; and/or
- he has a strong faith in God; and/or
- he's able to be accurate and objective when sick; and/or
- he has a good attitude despite being sick; and/or
- he generally has a strong immune system that fights illness; and/or
- he has a personality that is generally "up"; and/or
- he generally shows emotional stability.

Can you tell when your teen is really not feeling well? How does he deal with illness? How does he communicate about his symptoms? Is your teen a Silent Sufferer, a Hypochondriac, a Strong One, or another category altogether? There may be several factors that contribute to your teen's varying responses to sickness. In any case, it's important to encourage your child to express his thoughts and feelings. You can validate your teen's feelings by giving him your undivided attention followed by strong reassurance. It's normal for both younger and older teens to have a general concern for their health, but if a teen begins to show signs of hypochondriasis, it may be a sign of a deeper emotional problem.

I remember when I was a teenager. I would attend a full day of school, have a strenuous volleyball practice, study until 11:00PM or 12:00AM, and get up the next morning at 6:30AM only to find myself doing the same routine all over again! Although I felt tired, my body seemed to recover quickly. My teen years continued in this mode. Consequently, stress and a lack of sleep became a consistent lifestyle for me.

Observe your teen's sleep habits by answering the following questions:

- Does your teen have a regular bed time on school nights? Yes / No

- Does your teen consistently go to bed before midnight?
  Yes / No / I don't know

- Does your teen consistently go to bed before 10:00PM? Yes / No / I don't know

- On Saturday mornings, does your teen consistently sleep in past 11:00AM? Yes / No / I don't know

- Does your teen complain about always being tired? Yes / No / I don't know

Many active teenagers do not think that they need much rest. They "burn the candle at both ends" and seem to keep on going. Young people often think that failing to get adequate sleep and rest will not really hurt them because they do not experience the consequences immediately. The fact is, however, that without adequate sleep and rest, the body will slowly weaken to the point of becoming prey to illness. The consequences of a lack of sleep and rest, however, can and do appear later in life. If teens don't realize the connection between sufficient sleep and good health, their busy, stressed-filled habits will simply become a lifestyle when they become adults.

I am now 34 years old, and my medical doctor tells me that he cannot prescribe a medication to treat my uncomfortable physical symptoms that I have been experiencing for many years because they do not come under any specific diagnostic category. Since my doctor has not been able to help me, and since I'm "sick and tired" of feeling "sick and tired," I've begun to investigate alternative health sources. In my search to strengthen my body, I've noticed a profound connection between sleep and my overall physical health. Dr. Swank, a specialist in the treatment of multiple sclerosis says, "Sleep and adequate rest are like making a deposit in the bank for our health later." Teens, as well as adults, need to start making "sleep deposits" into their own good health bank accounts.

Teenagers' bodies are constantly changing. Their hormones are in high gear and their emotions are on a roller coaster. Without sufficient sleep, this already difficult time can become overwhelming. Furthermore, a lack of sleep can also contribute to a communication barrier between teens and their parents as teens become too "grumpy" or "edgy" to talk.

Research has found that the best sleep occurs before the hour of midnight. If teens go to bed at 12:00AM and get up at 8:00AM, they would not receive the same quality of sleep as they would if they went to bed at 10:00PM and got up at 6:00AM. Although they would clock in the same number of hours of rest, they would not receive the same health benefit in return.

It's also true that it's better for the body to maintain a consistent sleeping pattern. Even if you're unable to get your teenager to go to bed at exactly the same time each night, consistently try to have him get up at or near the same time every morning.

# 3 Talk with Your Teen

Prevention is the best medicine. This belief is more than a theory; it's a fact. Personally benefiting from this fact usually requires a change in our lifestyle. If you find that your teen is not motivated to begin to live a life of prevention, spend more time with him. Explain the connection between the health of his physical body and his emotional, mental, and spiritual states. Every aspect of a teen's life needs attention. This is also true for adults. After reading all of the following questions, choose which ones would be the most effective ways for you to use to begin a casual conversation with your teen. Remember that your purpose is to get your teen to open up — not shut down as a result of you dominating the conversation.

Ask your teen the following questions to help start a conversation concerning disease prevention.

- *"How many hours of sleep do you think your body needs to maintain good health?"*

- *"How do you feel after you don't get enough sleep?"*

- *"How do you think sleep or lack of sleep affects your body's ability to fight sickness?"*

- *"What can a teenager do to help his/her body fight illness?"*

- *"What kind of patient do you think you are when you're not feeling well?"*

- *"What are your feelings about going to the doctor or hospital?"*

- *"Is there anything about sickness that you fear?"*

- *"How would you feel if you found out you had a serious disease?"*

## *Building a Strong Immune System*

The human body is a complex and remarkable creation. God equipped the human body with its own built-in armor to war against sickness and disease. We call the body's natural resistance network its immune system. A healthy body is a strong defense against illness.

"Good health, like bad health, begins at the cellular level. Healthy bodies produce special killer T-cells that constantly roam the system looking out for foreign invaders; attacking and destroying them when encountered. Few of us realize how many foreign invaders there are. Our bodies are under constant attack from chemicals, pollutants, pesticides, additives, free radicals, and more. Our protective cells must continuously identify and rid us of these potentially lethal invaders. In order to keep up with this monumental task, all of our cells need the best of care."[17]

Have you ever heard the comment, "Some bug is going around. It just seems like everyone in school is getting hit with the same illness?" Doctors call times like these flu seasons. This typically occurs when people are together in close quarters and remain indoors most of the time due to the weather. After being around individuals who are carrying germs, students carry these viruses home to their families where the illness is spread to the other members.

Why is it that some people never get sick during the flu season? People who don't seem to "catch" the bugs may have developed an immunity in their bodies to that virus or bacteria. The development of this acquired immunity is called the immune response. When the body is invaded by a foreign substance the lymphocytes are triggered to produce special proteins called antibodies. If the body's resistance is strong enough, the antibodies eventually destroy the pathogen. From that time on, one's lymphocytes have made a mental note of the germ and can destroy it quickly if it reappears.

The main factors that contribute to an individual's strong immune system are:

- adequate sleep,
- proper nutrition,
- enough pure, clean drinking water,

- appropriate supplements,
- lack of allergies (food or otherwise),
- minimum negative stress (mental, emotional, or physical),
- proper exercise,
- recreational "fun" outlets,
- healthy relationships, and
- positive attitudes.

All of these factors play an important role in the function of the body at the cellular level. When the cells are healthy and operating at peak performance, there is less chance of them being overtaken by an illness. If your teen seems to be easily susceptible to colds or the flu, evaluate the previous list of factors to see where your teen may need a change.

##  Take Action

When making observations concerning your teen's health, you may sometimes feel that you are unable to remedy the situation by yourself. The following Action Steps, however, will help you make practical sense of your observations. They should help you to incorporate prevention into your teen's life.

- Place your teen in one of the following categories:
    - ❏ The Silent Sufferer
    - ❏ The Hypochondriac
    - ❏ The Strong One
    - ❏ Other or combination of the above:_____

- In light of how you categorized your teen, how might you communicate better with your teen when he/she is sick?


- After reading this section on infectious diseases, do you think that your teen shows signs of having a weakened immune system? Yes / No/ I don't know

- If your teen has a weakened immune system, place a check in the box of the main factors you feel are contributing to this condition:
  - ❏ lack of adequate sleep
  - ❏ lack of proper nutrition
  - ❏ lack of enough pure, clean drinking water
  - ❏ lack of appropriate supplements
  - ❏ possible food or other allergies
  - ❏ too much mental, emotional, and/or physical stress
  - ❏ lack of proper exercise
  - ❏ lack of recreational "fun" outlets
  - ❏ lack of healthy relationships, and
  - ❏ lack of healthy attitudes.

- Record the three items from the list above that you feel have the greatest effect on your teen:

  - ■ _____

  - ■ _____

  - ■ _____

- How might you help your teen in the areas that affect him/her the most?


- Read a book together on nutrition.

- Relieve any unnecessary pressure that you may be placing on your child.

- Have more healthy snacks available around the house.

- Be more consistent on a regular bed time.

- Purchase supplements (vitamins and minerals).

- See a physician (medical doctor and/or naturopathic physician) for more help if your teen seems frequently sick or tired.

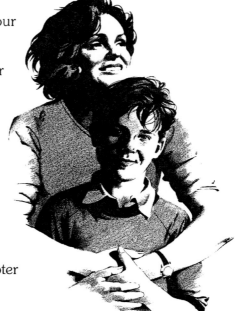

- Identify and resolve any conflicts in your teen's friendships.

- Identify and resolve any conflicts in your home.

- Other positive ideas: _____
  _____

- I'm interested in looking into a water purifying system or filter for our home.

## 5 Pause to Reflect

After you finish the appropriate Action Steps, complete this evaluation to see how the chapter worked for you.

- How well did you "connect" with your teen in this section?

  Not very well　　　Fairly well　　　Very well

- What did you learn about your teen's health that you did not know before this connection?

- What did you discover about your family's health patterns and habits as a result of this material?

- What did this chapter teach you about yourself?

- How successful were the Action Steps for your situation?

  Not successful          Somewhat successful          Very successful

- Record any further insights, questions, or comments concerning this section here:

## Further Resources

*Prescription for Nutritional Healing*, James F. Balch, M.D. and Phyllis A. Balch, (C.N.C. Avery Publishing Group, 1990). A comprehensive and up-to-date self-help guide. A practical A-Z reference to drug-free remedies using vitamins, minerals, herbs, and food supplements.

*None of These Diseases*, S.I. McMillen, M.D. (Fleming H. Revell, 1984). A physician testifies that health, happiness, and longer life can be yours if you follow the teachings of the Bible.

*The Natural Way to Vibrant Health*, Dr. N.W. Walker. (The Norwalk Press, 1972). Vibrant Health can only be realized by following a natural way of life eliminating artificial processed foods and by stimulating your mind and body through proper nutrition and thought.

*Diet and Salad*, Dr. N.W. Walker. (The Norwalk Press, 1971). A cook book as well as a nutritional guide; belongs in every homemaker's kitchen. The chemical elements in foods — protein, amino acids, milk starches, etc. are clearly explained. Dozens of recipes; entire menus help you plan healthful, nourishing meals.

*Become Younger*, Dr. N.W. Walker. (The Norwalk Press, 1978). The cornerstone of the famous Walker Program. What place has nutrition in the scheme of good health? How can the body and mind be so tuned that 'old age' might be defeated? Prepares you to take better care of your body.

*Juicing For Life*, Cherie Calbom and Maureen Keane. (Avery Publishing Group Inc., 1992). An excellent and comprehensive guide to the health benefits of fresh fruit and vegetable juicing.

*Total Health: Choices for a Winning Lifestyle*, Susan Boe, (RiversEdge Publishing, 1995). A comprehensive, easy-to-read high school textbook on health with relevant information including: Types of Fatigue, page 116; Stages of Sleep, page 118; Insomnia, page 120; Hints for Getting a Better Night's Sleep, page 120; The immune system, page 132–135; Fighting common infectious diseases *e.g.*, the common cold, pneumonia, mononucleosis, page 136–139.

# Sexually Transmitted Diseases, HIV, and AIDS

*In an effort to seem tolerant, the majority of doctors have taken a position of moral indifference toward their patients. The only reason they give for abstaining from sexual activity is the danger of venereal diseases or unwanted pregnancies. As far back as 1924, however, the Commission of Christian Social Morality recognized the insufficiency of fear as a deterrent for sexual promiscuity; for they wrote: "What is needed is not a mere unwillingness to perform the act, but a moral repudiation of it... to be satisfied with saying 'Avoid this, or you will suffer from it' is to stimulate ingenuity to find a means by which the consequences can be avoided."[18]*

*Sexually transmitted diseases (STDs) are a major health problem around the world. Medical science recognizes at least twenty-four different venereal diseases with scores of debilitating complications. The most common STDs are: chlamydia, gonorrhea, syphilis, herpes simplex II, and HIV which causes AIDS. It is important to communicate to your teen that condoms are no guarantee of protection against venereal disease. [19]*

## 1 Know the Causes

**Chlamydia** is one of the most common sexually transmitted diseases in the United States. It is estimated that between 3 to 10 million sexually active teenagers have contracted this disease. The signs of chlamydia include painful urination, unusual discharge from penis or vagina, and pain in the pelvic area. If untreated, this disease can cause permanent damage to the reproductive system. Since there is no natural immunity to chlamydia, a person can be infected a number of times.

**Gonorrhea** is a very common venereal disease. If left untreated, it can enter the rest of the body by way of the blood stream and affect the bones, joints, tendons, and other tissues. Gonorrhea is often undetected in females. If a female does experience symptoms, however, they would include frequent and painful urination, vaginal discharge, abnormal menstrual bleeding, inflammation of the pelvic area, and rectal itching. Symptoms for the male include yellow discharge from the penis and slow, difficult, and painful urination. Gonorrhea is often called the "preventer of life" because it can cause sterility in both males and females.

**Syphilis** is a sexually transmitted disease that has been called the "great imitator" because it looks like so many other diseases. This fact, however, does not make it less harmful. Syphilis is one of the least common but most dangerous venereal diseases. It can be contracted through kissing as well as through sexual intercourse. If left untreated, it will progress for years going through three stages. The first stage includes a canker or sore at the infection location. The second stage is a rash that appears in the mouth or genital area. If the disease enters the third stage, brain damage, hearing loss, heart disease, and blindness can occur.

**Herpes Simplex II** causes painful rashes and sores in and around the genital area. Once infected with this disease, it remains in the body. Although there is no cure, the symptoms may disappear and never return. A person may also experience recurring bouts with the virus. **Herpes Simplex I** is a virus that produces cold sores or blisters around the mouth. It is generally considered less serious, but it is highly contagious and there is no cure. Herpes Simplex I is not considered a sexually transmitted disease because it is not transmitted through sexual intercourse.

**HIV** is the virus that causes AIDS. HIV (human immunodeficiency virus) creates more fear and frustration than any other STD. AIDS (acquired immunodeficiency syndrome) is not itself a disease but the result of the HIV virus. Two undisputed facts stand out in all the research concerning AIDS:

- AIDS is fatal. There is no cure.
- AIDS can be prevented.

290,000 cases of AIDS have been reported in the United States. The first cases of AIDS were reported in 1981. Eleven years later, by the end of 1992, more than 250,000 Americans had developed full-blown AIDS and more than 170,000 had died — nearly three times more Americans than those who died in the Vietnam War.

The Department of Health and Human Services reports that one in every 250 Americans now has the AIDS virus, and the current rate of infection is one new case every 13 minutes.

A person is said to be HIV-positive when tests show that the person's body is producing antibodies to the retrovirus that causes AIDS. An infected person may be symptom-free for weeks, months, or years because the virus may not progress quickly. When the symptoms appear, the individual is then said to have AIDS.

Although it is listed as a sexually transmitted disease, HIV can also be spread by using infected IV needles used in drug use, shooting steroids, ear-piercing, or tattooing. Receiving infected blood products or being born to an infected mother are also ways of infection. HIV has been found in blood, semen, saliva, tears, nervous system tissue, breast milk, and vaginal fluids. To date, however, only semen and blood have been a proven means of infection.

In summary, a person can get AIDS from:

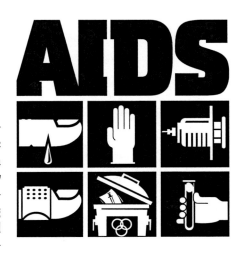

- sexual contact with an infected person,
- using an infected needle, and
- infected blood.

There is only one sure prevention of any sexually transmitted disease. The only true "safe sex" is no sex. That is why abstaining from sexual intercourse until marriage is not only pleasing to God, but a very wise health decision. Many pastors today are encouraging both partners to get blood tests for STDs and AIDS before marriage. Many states are requiring premarital blood testing to include the test for AIDS. Furthermore, faithfulness after marriage will continue to prevent STDs and AIDS.

## 2 Observe Your Teen

Every Christian parent would like to train his/her children in moral purity and godly living. Making wise choices in every area of life is our desire for our teens. Unfortunately, our best intentions are still up to the free will of our children. Even "the best laid plans of mice and men go awry," as Shakespeare keenly observed.

Even after receiving parental love, discipline, and instruction, teens will still make their own choices and receive the consequences. I have witnessed the devastating effects on parents when their teen steps out from under their guidance and makes an unwise decision. With the "Father heart of God" as our example we, too, can have mercy and grace for our children. He enables us to pour out our love upon a repentant child.

The goal of this observation section is to find out what your child knows about STDs and to clarify any standard of moral abstinence he may have concerning premarital sex. Abstinence from premarital intercourse, however, should not be the only goal for our teenagers.[20] Unfortunately, many Christian young people still engage in sexual activity even though they do not have intercourse. They go "too far" without going "all the way."

Consider the following concerning your teen:

- Does your teen have a dating standard already established?
  Yes / No / I don't know

- Have you or your spouse spoken to your teen about STDs?
  Yes / No / I don't know

- If you have spoken to your teen about STDs, do they know the physical consequences of each disease? Yes / No / I don't know

- Does your teen know specifically how an STD can be spread?
  Yes / No / I don't know

- Has your teen ever expressed to you or your spouse a desire to remain a virgin until marriage? Yes / No / I don't know

- Does your teen know your standard on how far is "too far" concerning physical contact with the opposite sex? Yes / No / I don't know

- Do you allow your teen to go on single dates? (This would include activities that involved any pairing off into couples.)
  Yes / No / I don't know

- Does your teen express an interest in single-dating?
  Yes / No / I don't know

- If your teen does single-date, does he/she have a steady boy/girl friend?
  Yes / No / I don't know

Many teens are aware of the physical consequences of premarital sexual involvement. They know about the risk of contracting an STD, HIV, or having an unplanned pregnancy. Too many teens, however, often overlook the emotional and spiritual consequences. Some of the emotional consequences are based in the fact that both male and female teens enter relationships often looking for something completely different from what the other person wants or needs.

> "...boys' and girls' physical and emotional natures are different. Boys tend to respond in a much more physically demanding way than do girls. Girls tend to respond more to the emotional needs of security and closeness. Boys face a more physical want for sex, whereas girls face a more emotional desire for closeness and intimacy." [21]

With this difference in mind, imagine what can take place between two young people who have strong feelings toward one another. A young boy feels a strong physical desire for closeness while a young girl feels a strong emotional desire for closeness. If your son or daughter is in a pattern of single-dating, the opportunity for this "connection" is much more likely than if your teen does not practice single-dating.

You may confidently say to yourself, "I know my son or daughter has high moral standards and he/she believes strongly in abstinence before marriage." I want to reassure you that this is a great foundation, but just because a teen knows the right thing to do, it doesn't mean he/she will have the strength to overcome that temptation when the situation arises.

The previous application section was meant to educate your teen about the seriousness of STDs and help to bring a "connection" between you and your teen in the area of sexual issues. It should be a goal of every parent to develop such a healthy relationship with their teen that the teen feels confident coming to them to discuss concerns about his/her sexuality. (More in-depth conversation will take place in this area in the Social Unit of *The Parent Connection*).

## 3 Talk with Your Teen

"If you diligently heed the voice of the Lord your God and do what is right in His sight, give ear to His commandments and keep all his statutes, I will put none of these diseases on you which I have brought on the Egyptians. For I am the Lord who heals you." (Exodus 15:26)

Saying "no" to sexual involvement before marriage is the only true prevention of sexually transmitted diseases for a teenager. If after answering the observation questions you feel that you would like to engage in a deeper conversation with your teen concerning STDs, you may want to use the following Conversation Starters. As a reminder, you may find that an opportunity arises when you could share some of your own struggles when you were a teenager. Use wisdom and discretion when sharing, but remember that teens have a legitimate need to know that you understand their feelings and can really relate to them.

After reading all of the following questions, choose which ones would be the most effective ways for you to use to begin a casual conversation with your teen. Remember that your purpose is to get your teen to open up — not shut down as a result of you dominating the conversation.

- *"What are the ways that a person can contract a sexually transmitted disease?" (In light of this question, don't be afraid to ask your teen if he understands what intercourse is.)*

- *"Are you aware of anyone who has ever had a sexually transmitted disease?"*

- *"I was not aware of all the horrible symptoms and complications of sexually transmitted diseases. There are at least twenty four known STDs and they each have their negative effects on the body. Are you fearful of contracting an STD? How come?"*

- *"We hear a lot about "safe sex" these days. What do you think "safe sex" is?"*

- *"What is your feeling about abstinence from intercourse before marriage?"*

- *"In terms of physical involvement, what is going 'too far' for you?"*

- *"I know that you are aware of the physical consequences of sex before marriage. Do you think that there may also be any emotional or spiritual consequences from it?"*

- *"I heard the phrase 'technical virgin' the other day. Have you heard the term? What does it mean to you?"*

- *"If a single person makes a mistake and has sex before marriage, then marries a different person later in life, do you think this could have an effect on the couple's marriage? Why or why not?"*

- *"How would you feel about marrying someone who was not a virgin?"*

- *"What do you think are some reasons why a teen would have sex before marriage? Do you think the reasons are different for a boy than for a girl?"*

- *"Do you know anyone who has HIV? If you did, how would this make you feel and how might you treat this person?"*

- *"Why do you think it's important to set standards concerning your sexual behavior before you are confronted with a decision?"*

# 4 Take Action

When trying to get your teen to talk about his/her feelings concerning sexuality, you may feel awkward or uncomfortable. If a similar conversation has not occurred before this, it may seem too deep. Be flexible. Your teen will give you signs when he/she is open or closed to the subject. Don't push. Try again another time, and pray for an opportunity when it will seem more natural.

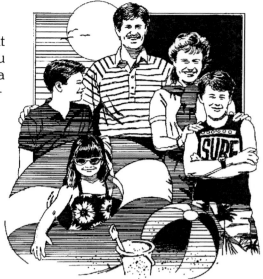

❏ After reading this section, do you feel that your teen has a conviction concerning abstinence? If so, what is that conviction?



❏ Do you feel your teen was just giving you the answers that he knew you wanted to hear, or were his comments genuine?

❏ Did your spouse get involved in the conversation? If so, how did it go? If not, do you think he/she should have another talk with your teen?



❏ Do you want to set aside a special "date" with your teen to discuss these issues and other issues that concern you?

Date with your teen:_____

Location:_____

❏ Dr. James Dobson, as well as some pastors, strongly recommend parents of teens buy a special bracelet or ring for their teen as a symbol of his/her commitment to virginity and moral purity. If interested, contact Focus on the Family for more details.

❏ Do you feel the need to talk with someone outside your family about these issues? If so, make a list of those to whom you are going to talk:

● _____

● _____

## *5* **Pause to Reflect**

After you finish the appropriate Action Steps, complete this evaluation to see how the chapter worked for you.

● How well did you "connect" with your teen about STDs?

Not well         Fairly well         Very well

● What did you learn about your teen that you did not know before this section?




● What did you discover about your family as a result of this chapter?




● What did this material teach you about yourself?




● How successful were the Conversation Starters with your teen?

Not successful        Somewhat successful        Very successful

● Record any further insights, questions, or comments concerning this section here:

## Further Resources

The Venereal Disease Hotline: 1–800–227–8922

The AIDS Hotline: 1–800–342–AIDS

Center For Disease Control

Focus on the Family
Colorado Springs, CO 80995–7451
1–800–A–FAMILY (1–800–232–6459)

*Preparing For Adolescence*, Dr. James Dobson. (Ventura, Regal Books, a Division of Gospel Light, 1989).

*None of These Diseases*, S.I. McMillen, M.D. (Fleming H. Revell, 1984). A physician testifies that health, happiness, and longer life can be yours if you follow the teachings of the Bible.

*How To Help Your Child Say "NO" To Sexual Pressure*, Josh McDowell. (Dallas: Word Publishing, 1987).

*RIGHT FROM WRONG: What You Need To Know To Help Youth Make Right Choices*, Josh McDowell and Bob Hostetler. (Dallas: Word Publishing, 1994).

*Talking With Your Kids about the Birds and the Bees*, Scott Talley. (Ventura, Regal Books, a division of Gospel Light Publications, 1987).

*Love, Sex, and God*, Bill Ameiss and Jane Graver. (Concordia Publishing House, 1982).

*Pure Excitement*, Joe White, (Focus on the Family Publishing, 1996).

# Noninfectious Diseases

*Although the human body is the most wonderful creation of all living things, it is not without its weaknesses. No matter how hard people may try to produce a perfect body through physical and mental training, the inner workings of the body are imperfect – there is no perfect "10!"* [22]

When Adam and Eve sinned in the Garden, the process of spiritual and physical degeneration began. Webster defines degeneration as: a lowering of effective power, vitality, or essential quality to a worsened kind or state; to pass from a higher to a lower type or condition. As a result of sin, Adam and Eve's relationship with God changed as did their mental and physical conditions.

## 1  Know the Causes

Scientists study noninfectious (noncommunicable) diseases to try to prevent them from occurring. Unlike infectious diseases (those that are caused by germs that spread from one person to another), three factors cause noninfectious diseases:

1. heredity,
2. environment, and
3. lifestyle.

Noninfectious diseases are said to be degenerative diseases because the body's tissues break down and do not grow or function properly. Although symptoms of a noninfectious disease may appear suddenly, the disease itself may have been developing over a long period of time. Most noninfectious diseases are called "chronic" because these illnesses can last over a long period of time. For this reason, prevention is very important in fighting degenerative diseases.

Modern medicine has a specific role in the fight against degenerative diseases. There is, however, a strength within the human body to restore itself. God has made the physical body with wonderful restorative abilities. The body is equipped to repair itself, and, with proper care, it can keep functioning properly. As you read the Observations section in this segment, you may develop some questions concerning yourself and/or your family's health, your environment, and/or your family's lifestyle. You may need to do some more personal research to answer all of your questions. When trying to prevent noninfectious diseases, such research is very important in order to form a full picture of the individual under consideration.

## 2 Observe Your Teen

### *Hereditary observations*

- Check any of the diseases listed below that your teen's biological father has in his health history:
  - ❏ heart disease
  - ❏ diabetes mellitus
  - ❏ hypoglycemia
  - ❏ high blood pressure
  - ❏ obesity
  - ❏ cancer
  - ❏ arthritis
  - ❏ cystic fibrosis
  - ❏ muscular dystrophy
  - ❏ multiple sclerosis

- Check any of the following diseases that your teen's biological mother has in her family history:
  - ❏ heart disease
  - ❏ diabetes mellitus
  - ❏ hypoglycemia
  - ❏ high blood pressure
  - ❏ obesity
  - ❏ cancer
  - ❏ arthritis
  - ❏ cystic fibrosis

❑ muscular dystrophy
❑ multiple sclerosis
❑ epilepsy

## *Environmental observations*

- Check any environmental factors that may contribute to the possibility of your teen developing a degenerative disease later in life:
  ❑ living near a main pollution source
  ❑ drinking impure water
  ❑ having a toxic occupation or job site
  ❑ living under/near large electrical power station or wires

- Check any lifestyle habits that may contribute to the possibility of your teen developing a degenerative disease later in life:
  ❑ tobacco use (smoking or chewing)
  ❑ extreme stress in his/her life
  ❑ obesity
  ❑ alcohol use
  ❑ lack of adequate exercise
  ❑ lack of proper nutrition
  ❑ improper sleeping habits
  ❑ consuming large amounts of salt
  ❑ the tendency to keep emotions and frustrations inside
  ❑ high fat/cholesterol diet

- Does your teenage daughter know how to give herself a proper breast examination? Yes / No / I don't know

- Does your teenage son know about testicular cancer, and is he able to give himself a testicular examination? Yes / No / I don't know

- Are you concerned about the future health of your teen because of the habit(s) he/she has begun? (If so, which one(s)?)
  Yes / No / I don't know

- Would you like to learn more about the prevention of degenerative diseases? Make a note of which disease(s) concern you.
  Yes / No / I don't know

- Does your teenager have mood swings based on what he does or does not eat? Does he complain about being weak and shaky when he does not eat? If so, do you think that your teen may have a blood sugar problem such as hypoglycemia? If you are concerned about the possibility, please see your medical doctor. Yes / No / I don't know

- Does your teenager urinate frequently, feel thirsty much of the time, and have increased appetite with unexplained weight loss? Has he experienced unexplained vomiting or nausea, general weakness, or fatigue? If so, do you think that your teen may have a blood sugar problem such as diabetes? If you are concerned about the possibility, please see your medical doctor.
  Yes / No / I don't know

## 3 Talk with Your Teen

After answering the preceding Observation questions, you may feel the need to engage in a deeper level of communication with your teen about degenerative disease. If so, you may wish to use the following Conversation Starters. At the beginning of any discussion of degenerative diseases, it's always good to refer to a family health history because it gives your teen a clear point of reference. Being able to say to your teen, "You had an uncle who died at age 45 from a heart attack" will be much more meaningful than citing the fact that heart disease is the number one killer in the United States. After reading all of the following questions, choose which ones would be the most effective ways for you to use to begin a casual conversation with your teen. Remember that your purpose is to get your teen to open up — not shut down as a result of you dominating the conversation.

- *"Do you know anyone who is diabetic? If so, how is their life different from yours? What is the primary concern of someone who has diabetes?"*

- *"Do you know anyone who has cancer? If so, how has their life, and their family's life, been affected by the disease?*

- *"When someone speaks about cancer how does it make you feel?"*

- *"Why do you think that heart disease is called the 'silent killer'?"*

- *"How do you think that teenagers can begin to make positive choices to help them in the prevention of heart disease?"*

- *"If your best friend's mother was diagnosed with cancer, how might you talk with your friend?"*

- *"What are some of the risks that teens take that may increase their risk of degenerative diseases?"*

- *"If your father had a serious heart attack and the doctor told him to change his lifestyle, what do you think those changes would consist of?"*

## 4 Take Action

After using the Conversation Starters to talk with your teen, you may feel that you need to take some specific steps of action concerning the prevention of degenerative disease in your family. The following activities and suggestions are intended to increase awareness of the need for personal change and provide some practical steps on how to implement it.

❏ **Specify your concern.** What is your primary concern for your teen's health concerning the risk of developing a degenerative disease?

- hereditary
  more specifically: _____.

- environment
  more specifically: _____.

- lifestyle
  more specifically: _____.

❏ **Write a tribute to a friend.** If your teen has had a close friend or relative pass away or is alive but sick with a serious illness, have them write a tribute to that person.

❏ **Do a health history family tree.** This is an activity that your teen's health teacher may assign in class. If your teen does not receive this as a class assignment, it would be lots of fun to do as a family project and well worth the

time. It would involve you and your spouse doing a complete and thorough job of family research.

❏ **Visit the family doctor together.** It would be a great example to your teen if you and your spouse were to get full physical examinations. Then the family could work together to prevent any risks of disease that may be mentioned.

❏ **Do research in the following areas** as they relate to your family health history and your concern for your teen's health:

● cancer
● diabetes
● epilepsy
● obesity-related diseases
● heart disease
● high blood pressure
● cholesterol
● multiple sclerosis
● muscular dystrophy
● cystic fibrosis

● other: _____

## *5* Pause to Reflect

After you finish the appropriate Action Steps, complete this evaluation to see how the chapter worked for you.

● How well did you "connect" with your teen in this section?
 Not very well     Fairly well     Very well

● After reading this section, do you feel that your teen takes his/her good health for granted? Yes / No / I don't know

- Do you feel that your teen thinks or feels that he is indestructible much of the time? Yes / No / I don't know

- Do you feel that your teen is overly worried that he will contract a degenerative disease? Yes / No / I don't know

- What did you learn about your own health history that you did not know before?

- What did you discover about your spouse's health history that you did not know before?

- How successful were the Action Steps in your situation?
  Not successful        Somewhat successful        Very successful

- Record any further insights, questions, or comments concerning this section and your teen here:

## Further Resources

*Healthy Living in a Toxic World*, Cynthia Fincher, Ph.D. (Pinon Press, 1996).

*Alzheimer's, Caring for Your Loved One, Caring For Yourself*, Sharon Fish. (Harold Shaw Publishers, 1990).

*Damaged But Not Broken, A Personal Testimony of How to Deal with the Impact of Cancer*, Larry Burkett, (Moody Press, 1996).

*Prescription for Nutritional Healing*, James F. Balch, M.D. and Phyllis A. Balch. (C.N.C. Avery Publishing Group, 1990). A comprehensive and up-to-date self-help guide. A practical A-Z reference to drug-free remedies using vitamins, minerals, herbs, and food supplements.

*None of These Diseases*, S.I. McMillen, M.D. (Fleming H. Revell, 1984). A physician testifies that health, happiness, and longer life can be yours if you follow the teachings of the Bible.

*The Natural Way to Vibrant Health*, Dr. N.W. Walker. (The Norwalk Press, 1972). Vibrant Health can only be realized by following a natural way of life eliminating artificial processed foods and by stimulating your mind and body through proper nutrition and thought.

*Diet and Salad*, Dr. N.W. Walker. (The Norwalk Press, 1971). A cook book as well as a nutritional guide; belongs in every homemaker's kitchen. The chemical elements in foods — protein, amino acids, milk starches, etc. are clearly explained. Dozens of recipes; entire menus help you plan healthful, nourishing meals.

*Become Younger*, Dr. N.W. Walker. (The Norwalk Press, 1978). The cornerstone of the famous Walker Program. What place has nutrition in the scheme of good health? How can the body and mind be so tuned that 'old age' might be defeated? Prepares you to take better care of your body.

*Juicing For Life*, Cherie Calbom and Maureen Keane. (Avery Publishing Group Inc., 1992). An excellent and comprehensive guide to the health benefits of fresh fruit and vegetable juicing.

*Home Medical Encyclopedia*, The American Medical Association, Charles Clayman, (ed.). New York, (The Reader's Digest Association, Inc., with permission of Random House, Vols. 1–2).

# The Reproductive Systems and Human Sexuality

(Abstinence and dating issues will be covered in more detail in the Social Unit of ***The Parent Connection***)

*The problem today in the Christian community and especially with parents is there has been a conspiracy of silence when it comes to this area of human life. We of all people as Christians ought to have a firm good grip on the truth because our God created sexuality in the first place.*[23]

*The Parent Connection* has two goals relative to sex education. First, it is to help break the silence barrier in your home over this much-neglected subject. Second, it is to boost your confidence level in successfully addressing this area. (A more detailed section on the subject on forming a proper sexual identity will be discussed in the Social Unit). This section of *The Parent Connection* is organized differently than other chapters and will address the following areas:

- Overcoming barriers to communication about sex
- Common questions teens have about sex
- Tips for improving communication skills in the area of sex education
- Information about reproduction and contraception

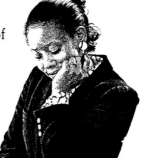

> "I always thought I would be different from my own parents... but I feel as uncomfortable as they did talking with my kids about sex."

One of the most difficult and probably one of the most controversial issues facing parents is the subject of sex education. As parents, we can learn both positives and negatives from our own upbringing. I think *every* generation has had a certain difficulty communicating about the subject of sexuality. It is difficult enough to talk about everyday subjects, let alone sexual topics with our children. Before discussing this subject, I tell my students that it is normal and natural to feel uneasy when discussing the organs and functions of the human reproductive systems. God has given each of us an inborn, godly modesty. This feeling of uneasiness causes people to respect one another's privacy. I also share with my students my belief that it is vital that their parents be the primary sex educators in their lives; not their friends, classmates, or the media.

It is interesting to note the following percentages that are the result of a survey done where teens were asked where they received most of their information about sex:[24]

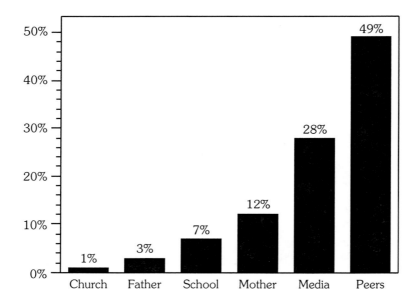

## *Overcoming Barriers to Communication About Sex*

Many parents want to have open communication with their teen concerning sexual issues. Many feel that it is their responsibility to do so, but they just don't know how. Why is it so difficult for parents and teens to talk with each other about sex? Dennis Rainey, in his tape series *Teaching Your Children About Sex*, lists seven barriers: [25]

1. **Improper perspective:** Your own view of sexuality may be unbiblical or unhealthy; overly-indulgent or prudish.

2. **Incorrect modeling:** How did your own parents teach you about sex? The temptation is to copy what and how we were taught as children. Determine that you are going to do a better job than your parents.

3. **Adult sexual sin:** You may feel ashamed or embarrassed about sex because you have not properly processed your own past sexual failures or because you are presently struggling with a sexual addiction or an affair.

4. **Shame:** Some parents fear that some of their own adolescent sexual failures will come to light in the discussion, and they are too ashamed to admit them.

5. **Insecurity:** Parents are often unsure of what information to tell and how much of it to tell. You may fear that you will say too much or say too little. You may dread making a mistake in communicating about sexual issues.

6. **Fear:** You may fear that the knowledge you give your teen may lead them to promiscuity.

7. **No agenda:** Some parents just don't have a clue at where to start and have no plan as to how and when to share what level of information.

## *Other Barriers Include:*

- Parents are concerned about telling too much about sex will only peek curiosity and make their teen want to experiment.

- Some teens are embarrassed to bring up the subject with their parents or feel guilty about having sexual thoughts.

- Many children feel anxious when their parents first bring up the subject of sex. To try to hide their anxiety, they respond to the topic as if they are completely bored.

- Parents and children may have difficulty seeing each other as individuals with sexual needs and desires.

- Many teens feel they already "know it all."

- Many parents believe that if their child has a question, he will take the initiative to bring it up himself.

- Many parents leave the discussion and the information up to the school, church youth group, or peers.

- Many parents give one or two "talks" concerning sex and sexuality and do not continue the education process in a natural way.

All of these hindrances are very real, but they can be overcome. If it is handled properly, the issue of sex is the single most powerful issue that opens up teens to the input of their parents. Healthy sex education in the home first requires a strong relational foundation between parent and child. This relationship begins at an early age.

My first experience with sex education as a student in school came in sixth grade when the boys and girls were split and our teacher showed the girls slides on the female menstrual cycle. At the end of the slide presentation, the teacher got up in front of the class with a red face and asked, "Are there any questions?" Before any of us could get up the nerve to ask a question, our teacher inserted, "Good," and then changed the subject.

What a disappointing introduction to sex education. In the context of learning and education, when is having no questions ever "good?" For whatever reason, questions are usually a very good sign that a student is beginning to process the information that he is learning. I'm afraid that my sixth grade teacher's insertion was only her own defense mechanism which actually blocked our learning. Whether it was out of ignorance, insecurity, fear, or embarrassment she didn't want us to ask her any questions about sex. Later, when I was in charge of my own health class discussion of sex, I allowed the girls to ask me questions. Openly hearing their questions gave me the opportunity to have many meaningful discussions with them which probably would not have occurred otherwise.

## Common Questions Teens Have About Sex

I was surprised at some of the questions that teenagers have about sexuality. You may be surprised, too, as you read the following list of teen questions. The following questions I have heard either in class or in counseling sessions with teenagers. You may wish to postpone some or all of these questions to the time of pre-marital counseling. But, that may not be possible. It would be ideal if these sexual subjects never entered their minds until they were engaged to get married. The majority of these questions are probably very similar to the ones that your own teen has on his/her mind right now.

Although the following questions were raised during a split class, the boys' questions are mixed in with the girls' questions.

- "Can I get pregnant from French kissing?"

- "I feel like I have appendicitis about once a month with pain on my side? What does this mean?"

- "What does it mean when my underwear gets wet?"

- "My Mom told me when I started my period that I could now get pregnant. So, is it true that if I have sex during my period then I can get pregnant?"

- "Do married couples have intercourse while the wife has her period?"

- "Why is it that God gave teenagers such strong sex drives but tells them that they can't fulfill these desires until later when they get married?"

- "If I don't experience nocturnal emissions (wet dreams) does that mean I am not normal?"

- "My breasts are tender about once a month and I feel lumps in them. I am afraid I might have breast cancer."

- "Is masturbation right or wrong?"

- "I have been curious about how homosexuals have sex. Does this mean I might be a homosexual?"

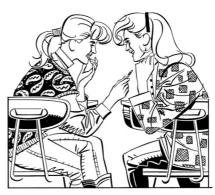

- "Is oral sex the same as French kissing?"

- "It seems like I bleed a lot during my period. How much is normal? Should I be concerned?"

- "I have horrible cramps during my period while some of my friends don't experience any discomfort. It isn't fair. Is there anything I can do about it?"

- "Why don't boys get 'periods'?"

- "How old do you have to be to start having sex?"

- "Does intercourse hurt?"

- "When does a boy's body start making sperm?"

- "Why is it so difficult to talk to my parents about sex?"

- "If sex is so great, why is it so wrong for us to do it before marriage?"

- "Why can't guys seem to control themselves more sexually?"

- "Why are guys who sleep around considered 'studs', but girls who do the same considered 'sleazy'?"

- "What was your honeymoon like?"

Being a good sex educator at home is more than just giving your children facts on reproduction and pregnancy. Children need to know that their questions are not stupid. They need to get the message from you that their feelings and thoughts on sexuality are natural and normal. What parents want to avoid are feelings of shame, guilt, or thoughts that sex is dirty. What parents want to impart to their teens is the fact that sex is a wonderful gift from God. He created it for two purposes: reproduction and pleasure.

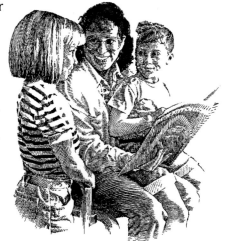

Even though you may have strong personal feelings about certain sexual subjects, try not to be surprised or judgmental when discussing sexual issues with your teen. Often, the best you can do is to listen to their questions or opinions. Your children will be more apt to listen to your opinion and values if you first listen to theirs.

Some teens get "misinformation" from peers, society, and the media. It is your responsibility to correct this misinformation and educate your teen correctly. For example, have you noticed your teen watching Soap Operas? Has she become so wrapped up in the lives of these stars that she does not really have a grasp on what real love is like? Unrealistic expectations in the minds of adults, as well as teens, can hinder otherwise healthy friendships. Romance novels and teen magazines can dramatize sex and romance to a devastating, unrealistic level.

## Tips For Improving Communication Skills in the Area of Sex Education

*We should not be ashamed to discuss what God was not ashamed to create.* [26]

The following suggestions may help you to communicate more effectively with your teen:

1. **Be approachable.** It is important to let your teen know that he will not be judged, teased, or punished for asking questions about sexuality. When you are approachable it sends a message to your teen that you understand and respect their curiosity about sex. It is also important for you not to wait for them to ask all of the questions. If you bring up the subject first, it will subconsciously give them permission to do the same. You may want to use your own adolescent experiences to help explain or bring up certain subjects. Share only as much as you feel your teen is ready to hear.

2. **Know the facts.** It would be a good idea for you to study the illustrations and materials in this section. They would serve as an excellent information update for you. Do not be surprised if your teen knows these words and definitions better than you. If you don't know the answer to a question, it is better to admit your ignorance and give them the correct answer after you search it out. Teens respect honesty.

3. **Avoid preaching.** When your child begins to ask questions about sex, and you have the opportunity to quote scripture to support your values, do it in a manner that is non-judgmental. Avoid talking "down" to your teen. Teens feel that when they are brave enough to ask questions about adult subject matter, they want to be treated like adults. If interest is there, a good Bible study on purity or morality would be appropriate.

4. **Be slow to speak.** It is tempting to interject your own ideas when your child is trying to form his thoughts or choice of words. It is also tempting to attempt to complete your teen's sentences for him because you know him so well or because he is somewhat slow at bringing out his thoughts. This is a great time just to listen. You may be surprised at how much insight you can gain when you just give your child your ear and not your opinion. Listen carefully for hidden messages when your teen asks a question or brings up a specific subject. For example, if your teenage daughter tells you that she recently learned about breast cancer in class, she may want to discuss her fears about the disease with you.

5. **Look for teachable moments.** A teachable moment is an unplanned and unexpected opportunity when your child becomes emotionally open to discuss issues or receive information. A TV commercial containing a strong sexual message is a good example of a teachable moment, a natural opportunity for the discussion of sexual issues. A story on the evening news or an article in the newspaper may also be used to prompt relevant discussion. When such teachable moments occur, you can ask your child several questions. First, what message is really being sent here? Second, is the message realistic or idealistic (and, therefore, ultimately deceptive)? Third, what is someone trying to sell? Fourth, how does the advertisement make you feel?

6. **Openly discuss peer pressure.** The influence of peers is the strongest influence for teenagers. You can help your teen deal with sexual peer pressure by pointing out the following:

- Even though it may seem like it, not everyone is "doing it."

- Having a sexual relationship or even having a boyfriend or girlfriend will not solve the problems of growing up.

- Having sexual intercourse does not transform a teen into an adult — waiting until marriage is the true test of maturity.

- Having sexual intimacy is not a proof of true love.

- Refusing to be sexually active does not make a person a "prude" or a homosexual.

- A man will never physically hurt his body if he doesn't have intercourse.

- Having a relationship or dating someone steadily does not always equal "fun."

- The media and peers do not explain all of the spiritual, emotional, and relational pain associated with pre-marital sexual involvement.

7. **Communicate your values in love.** You can help your teen establish her own sexual values as you communicate — and live out — your own beliefs about sexual behavior in a kind way. It won't work to try to force your teen to adopt your personal convictions. As a matter of fact, parents who try to dictate what their teen should believe when the teen has not consistently and voluntarily integrated those values into her own life, will find that their teen will most likely rebel and reject those values.

8. **Respond with understanding and love if your teen makes a mistake.** The phrase, "What my parents don't know won't hurt them," is often used when kids "mess-up" and feel that they can't tell their parents. I would rather have my child come to me and tell me his mistakes rather than to have him not trust whether my response will be one of love and forgiveness or not. When a parent can intervene with love and understanding it helps to stop the continuing progression of the poor choices. It also shows the heart of our heavenly Father. He wants us all to come to Him so He can help us overcome our temptations rather than to hide our mistakes and try to "go it alone."

## *Information About Reproduction and Contraception*

The following information is a brief overview of reproduction. Having just one conversation with your child about reproduction is never enough. It takes more than one sex education "talk" with your child to communicate information as well as values.

Children misunderstand, forget information, and come up with more questions.

The female reproductive system, listed from the outside to the inside of the body, includes: the vulva, the labia, the clitoris, the urethra, the vagina, the cervix, the uterus, the fallopian tubes, and the ovum (or, egg).

**Definition of terms:**

- The **vulva** is the area between a woman's legs that leads to the vagina.

- The two sets of lips that make up the vulva are called the **labia**. As a girl matures, the outer lips will grow pubic hair in order to protect the body.

- The **clitoris** is the place where the inner lips meet. It is a very small and sensitive area above the vaginal opening which plays a vital role in female sexual arousal.

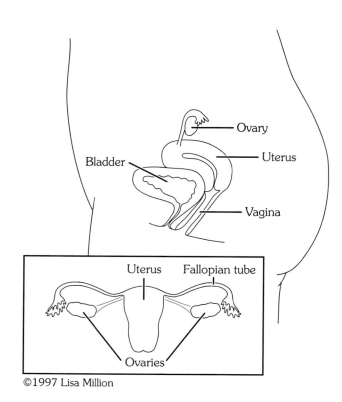

©1997 Lisa Million

- The **urethra** is the urinary opening. It is often the source of infection if a woman does not keep herself cleansed properly.

- The **vagina** is the canal that stretches from the outside of the body to the cervix.

- The **cervix** is a small cylindrical organ, an inch or so in length and less than an inch in diameter. It makes up the lower part of the neck of the uterus. The cervix separates the body and cavity of the uterus from the vagina.

- The **uterus** (or, womb) is a small, muscular sac that provides a place for the fertilized egg to grow and develop. During pregnancy the size of the uterus expands to many times its original size. After delivery, the uterus will slowly decrease in size again.

- The **fallopian tubes** are the two narrow passageways from each of the ovaries to the uterus. Each month one egg travels to the uterus through one of the fallopian tubes.

- An **egg** (or, ovum) is the reproductive cell supplied by the female which is released from one of the two ovaries each month.

- **Ovulation** is the process in which one ovary each month releases an egg that travels down the fallopian tube to the uterus. Some girls experience discomfort during ovulation. During the three to five days of a woman's cycle, she does not know for sure on what day her egg will travel. After an egg is released it can only live up to 24 hours. Technically speaking then, a woman can only become pregnant one day out of every month! If this is true, why do women get pregnant so often? The reason is because the male sperm can live up to 72 hours after being released in the woman's body.

The male reproductive system includes: the prostate gland, the testes, the scrotum, and the penis. Unlike the female reproductive system, most of the organs of the male system lie outside the male body.

**Definition of terms:**

- The **testicles** or **testes**, produce **testosterone**, the male hormone that triggers development of male secondary sex characteristics, such as facial

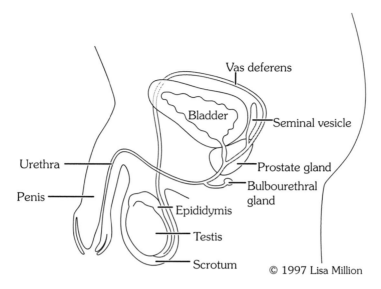

Vas deferens

Bladder

Seminal vesicle

Urethra

Prostate gland

Bulbourethral gland

Penis

Epididymis

Testis

Scrotum

© 1997 Lisa Million

hair and voice changes. After puberty, the testicles also continually produce **sperm**, the male reproductive cells.

- The **scrotum** is the sac that surrounds the testes. The scrotum lies outside the body to reduce the temperature of the testes.

- The **vas deferens** brings the sperms from the testes to the ejaculatory duct, where some sperm are stored temporarily.

- **Semen**, which is ejaculated from the penis, is made up of tiny sperm cells mixed with various fluids. An important fluid contained in the semen is fructose (sugar), which stimulates the sperm to become mobile and travel to meet the egg. Sperm can live up to 72 hours after being ejaculated.

- The **penis** is the organ that is used for urination and reproduction. It is composed of spongy tissues that contain small blood vessels and nerves.

- An **erection** occurs when an adolescent or adult male is sexually excited. A man's blood flow increases causing more pressure within the penis. As a result, the penis becomes long and hard.

- **Ejaculation** occurs when the erect penis releases semen. One ejaculation contains about one teaspoon full of semen which can contain up to 400 million sperm.

- **Nocturnal emissions** (or, "wet dreams") occur when the penis ejaculates semen when a male is asleep. This is a perfectly normal experience, and boys have no control over when it happens.

## *Pregnancy*

The male sperm cell is one of the smallest of all human cells. It carries the father's full legacy to the child. The female egg is much larger in comparison to the sperm. It carries the mother's full legacy to the child. During a male ejaculation, millions of sperm are released. While each sperm tries to swim vigorously toward the one female egg, only one sperm will successfully penetrate and fertilize the egg. When a sperm has penetrated the egg, the egg hardens and does not allow any other sperm to enter.

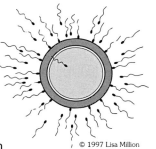

© 1997 Lisa Million

Ovulation is the time when an egg is released from an ovary and travels through a fallopian tube on its way to the uterus. Pregnancy can only occur during ovulation. **Conception** is the term used to describe the moment when an egg cell is fertilized by a sperm. After conception has occurred, the fertilized egg attaches itself to the uterus where it begins to grow.

## *Menstruation*

Every month the uterus prepares to support a fertilized egg. The lining of the uterus begins to thicken with blood to prepare for ovulation. If fertilization does not take place, the lining of the uterus breaks down and passes out of the female body. This process is called **menstruation**. If fertilization does take place during ovulation, the lining of the uterus is used to supply nourishment to the growing fetus which implants itself on the uterine wall. The amount of blood that is passed out of the female body and the length of time of menstruation varies among females. When all the tissue and blood is gone from the uterus, one of the ovaries begins to release another egg. The time from one menstruation to the next is called the menstruation

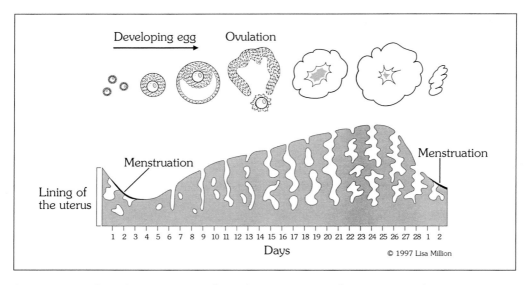

Developing egg  Ovulation

Menstruation

Menstruation

Lining of
the uterus

1 2 3 4 5 6 7 8 9 10 11 12 13 14 15 16 17 18 19 20 21 22 23 24 25 26 27 28 1 2

Days

© 1997 Lisa Million

(or, menstrual) cycle. The time of the female's blood flow is also referred to as her "period." Without the menstrual cycle, reproduction would not occur.

Some females experience varying degrees of discomfort during their menstrual cycle. This discomfort is called **premenstrual syndrome (PMS)**. PMS has been linked to food allergies, candidiasis, low blood sugar (hypoglycemia), malabsorption of nutrients, and hormonal imbalance — excessive estrogen levels and inadequate progesterone levels.[27]

Some of the physical discomforts of PMS may include:
- tender and swollen breasts
- cramping in the abdomen
- weakness and fatigue
- cravings for particular foods (chocolate, sweets, etc.)
- weight gain and feeling "fat"
- diarrhea or loose bowel movements
- nausea and vomiting
- headaches
- backache
- insomnia
- fainting spells

Some of the emotional discomforts of PMS may include:
- irritability
- emotional moodiness
- depression (slight to severe thoughts of suicide)
- outbursts of anger

The following are some recommendations to help alleviate the symptoms of PMS. The following should be done one to two weeks before a female's period is to begin. [28]

- Avoid salt, caffeine, alcohol, red meats, dairy products, sugar in any form, processed foods, junk foods, or fast foods.

- Do not smoke.

- Eat plenty of fresh fruits and vegetables, whole grains, cereals, breads, beans, peas, lentils, nuts, seeds, broiled chicken, turkey, and fish. Have high protein snacks between meals.

- Drink eight glasses of purified water a day.

- Consider taking one or more of the following supplements under the supervision of your healthcare provider:
  - ❏ calcium with magnesium chloride
  - ❏ primrose oil
  - ❏ vitamin B complex with extra $B_5$ and $B_6$

## Contraception

The subject of contraceptives is one of the most fear-ridden, confusing, and controversial issues in sex education. Christian parents and educators both struggle with the questions of if, when, and how much to explain to their teens about this issue. The two views that I most commonly hear from Christians are:

- Contraceptives should only be discussed in the context of premarital counseling.

- Contraceptives should be discussed with teens as they learn about abstinence.

Many factors can lead parents to discuss birth control with their teen. Some of them are in defensive reaction to what their teen has heard from other sources. What do you do if your teen hears about different contraceptives from the media or their peers? (The reason I have heard teens ask questions is because they heard about contraceptives somewhere and did not want to seem ignorant among their peers.) Or, what do you do if your son or daughter asked you what you and your husband use for the prevention of pregnancy? You must have a plan on what and how much you are going to share with your teen, even if your original plan is never to raise the subject yourself. If your child does raise a question, and you do not know how you want to handle it, just say, "That's a great question. Could you give me a few days, and I'll talk to you about it later?"

There are three main reasons why some Christian families feel that sex education for their teenager should address the subject of contraception:

1. The first reason that teenagers need some form of information about contraceptives is because of the way that they are being bombarded by the media and their peers with the propaganda of "safe sex." When parents discuss birth control with their teen, they have the opportunity to dispel this very prevalent myth among young people. The "safe sex" philosophy promotes the idea that premarital sex is OK just as long as the male uses a condom. As we know to the contrary, abstinence is the only safe sex. Abstinence is the only guaranteed way to prevent pregnancy, avoid sexually transmitted diseases, respect oneself and one's special friend, prepare for marriage, and please God.

2. The second reason is that Christian young people as a whole are much more promiscuous than most of us realize. Not only are more Christian teens engaging in sexual intercourse, but many are involved in sexually stimulating behaviors which they keep hidden from their parents. Much of this behavior, little doubt, is being influenced by the myth of "safe sex." Teaching absti-

nence is not sufficient in itself. If abstinence is taught at the exclusion of teaching on moral purity, then we can produce teens who may not go "all the way," but consistently go much "too far" in their dating relationships. The goal of teaching our teens the desirability of being virgins when they get married is correct, but let us not forget that sexual impurity in the New Testament is not just the constant thought of lust but consciously doing anything that sexually stimulates the other person outside the context of marriage.

3.  The third reason that some believe that contraception is a good topic to discuss with teens is because it is a great opportunity to increase their moral development when the subject of abstinence is addressed. We can spend a lot of time discussing whether birth control should or should not be discussed and how much information we should or should not tell our teens. Parents as well as educators can easily become so concerned about the physical aspects of sex education (trying to protect them from too much information) that we forget the main objectives of sex education (moral and spiritual development). Many times, what they have heard is information without character being attached to it; facts and statistics without what the Word says about sexuality.

4.  The fourth reason why some parents believe they should address the area of contraception is the sad but nevertheless true fact that some of our teens are going to choose to disobey God's law against premarital sex and do it anyway. I think this is a very difficult and uncomfortable thought. It is also interesting to note that if a teen were to use protection, does that mean that he/she was prepared because it was a pre-planned activity, and thus a worse offense than a moment of uncontrolled passion? This "judgement" leaves us something to think about. I know that all of us would rather not even think of our teen being in a morally compromising situation, but unfortunately it occurs. Scott Talley, a youth minister for 17 years and author of *Talking with your Kids about the Birds and the Bees*, helps parents put this delicate issue into realistic perspective:

    > "I would suggest that parents not dilute their own and God's view on sexual sins. Sex before marriage remains a sin. You should clearly communicate this fact to your teen. But, I also feel that teenagers can be told that, if they choose to violate parental and godly views, they should protect themselves and use contraceptives....I have not been able to find any evidence that [demonstrates that] providing birth control information to teenagers encourages sexual

activity...I am not advocating the distribution of contraceptives, [I am] merely [suggesting] the giving of knowledge and information....Christian teenagers engage in sexual activity because they have a low self-esteem, because they have poor relationships, either at home or with their peers, or because they have allowed themselves to be in a situation where physical contact is extremely difficult to control and they have succumbed to temptation. But I have never read, heard or seen any evidence that Christian teenagers have had sexual intercourse because they had knowledge of birth control or because it was available."[29]

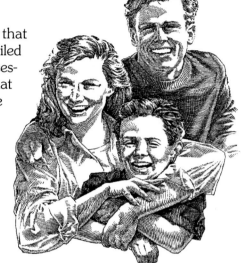

Please do not misunderstand me. I admit that there is a valid concern that too much detailed information too early may stimulate an unnecessary curiosity. We must always remember that the main objective in sex education should be to build moral character in our children so that they can understand their God-given sex drive, handle peer pressure, live a morally pure life, and learn self-control. Abstinence is not the only issue to be stressed in sex education. The root issue is to shape and mold the child's conscience. Sex education is a lifelong process. We want our children to grow up to be responsible teens who then grow up to become self-controlled, responsible adults! As Dennis Rainey puts it, "Minor on the biological aspects of sex, but major on the issues of character."[30]

If we major on the minors, we will miss the main objective of sex education.

The marriage bed today could be much better for a lot of couples if their parents would have taken the time to take the sex education of their children more seriously. The following are some ideas that may help:

1. Take personal responsibility for the sex education of your children.

2. Talk to your spouse about what was his/her source of sex education. Discuss the values — both healthy and unhealthy — associated with that source.

3. If you are a single parent, share with a close friend of the same gender about how you can develop a sex education plan for your children.

4. Admit your uneasiness with discussing this subject. All of us have a God-given shyness when it comes to sexuality for reasons of purity and privacy.

5. Incorporate the following categories into the sex education of your children:
   - A godly view of sexuality.
   - An understanding of their own sex drive and that of the opposite sex.
   - Principles by which they can build their own personal convictions.
   - A strong belief of who they are as children of God and temples of the Holy Spirit.
   - Teach the divine purposes of sex: [31]
     - to glorify God in our bodies
     - to reflect God in our sexual nature
     - to reproduce a godly heritage
     - to participate in a divine miracle
     - to enjoy a special intimacy

6. Set some goals and have a plan.

7. The plan is a process and is not necessarily the same for every family or family member.

8. Be willing to learn some principles as you go along.

You can get more information about contraceptives from the office of a gynecologist. If the subject of birth control does come up in your home a little earlier than you anticipated, you need not jump to the conclusion that your teen is sexually active. Curiosity — and the desire to know as much as their peers — plays a big role in a teen's desire for information concerning sexuality. It is great when a teen feels that his/her parents are the best source of information. The following information may help you be prepared as you form a plan of what you are going to say.

## Birth Control Methods

The following information is provided for you to use at your own discretion. The contraceptives that teens are most familiar with are: the condom, the pill, and natural planning (the "I-know-my-body" method).

### The Most Effective Birth Control Methods

- Abstinence:

Only abstinence offers 100% protection against unplanned pregnancy and STDs.

- Oral Contraceptives (the Pill):

The Pill is the most popular form of birth control in the United States (with the exception of sterilization). The Pill generally contains small doses of the female hormone estrogen and progestin (a progesterone-like substance), which prevent pregnancy primarily by preventing ovulation. Used correctly, the Pill is 99.9% effective. Some women, however, experience side effects such as bleeding between periods, breast tenderness, headaches, weight gain, and nausea. Today, teens may also be placed on the Pill by their gynecologist for various problems in their monthly cycle.

- The Intrauterine Device (IUD):

IUDs are T-shaped devices that are inserted into the uterus by a physician. The IUDs release either copper (this type may remain in place for up to 8 years) or progesterone (this type needs to be replaced once a year). Although IUDs are effective (97%) some women experience increased bleeding and pain during their menstrual cycle. The device also can become dislodged and cause problems within the uterus. There are two views concerning how the pregnancy is prevented. Some believe that the prevention occurs by way of an abortion by preventing implantation within the uterus. Others maintain that the use of an IUD produces an intrauterine environment that is spermicidal, and thus prevents fertilization.

- Contraceptive Implants:

Contraceptive implants consist of six hormone-filled rods inserted under the skin of the upper arm of the woman. They provide protection against pregnancy 24 hours a day for up to five years. Contraceptive implants have a high degree of effectiveness but also may cause irregular bleeding, decreased duration of the menstrual flow, or may actually cause amenorrhea (absence of menstruation).

- Hormonal Injection:

The hormonal injection, which must be prescribed by a doctor, contains a form of the hormone progesterone. Each injection provides protection for up to three months. This method has similar side effects to that of the Pill. After one year of use, as many as one-half of the women receiving the injections stop having their menstrual periods.

- Sterilization:

Sterilization is a permanent form of birth control. Women receive a tubal ligation which involves surgery on the fallopian tubes preventing any egg from being fertilized. Men receive a vasectomy which involves the cutting of the vas deferens which stops the passage of sperm to the penis.

**Barrier Methods**

- The Condom:

Condoms are the most widely discussed form of birth control, especially among teenagers. As a form of birth control, the condom has a 88% effectiveness rate. With correct and consistent use, the rate is 98%. Condoms are available with or without spermicide or lubricant and can be purchased without a prescription. Condoms gain attention in the area of "safe sex" because they may help in the prevention of STDs including HIV. Although condoms are one of the most commonly used forms of contraceptives among teenagers, inform your teen that their use does not guarantee "safe sex."

- The Diaphragm:

The diaphragm is a dome-shaped rubber cup that is filled with spermicide, inserted through the vagina, and set over the opening of the cervix. The diaphragm blocks the cervix so that no sperm can travel up into the fallopian tubes. The diaphragm must be prescribed by a doctor. It should not be left in place for more than 24 hours. The diaphragm must be used correctly to be effective. The effectiveness rate is as low as 82% because of the misuse of the device. The diaphragm may also cause an increase in urinary tract infections.

- The Cervical Cap:

The cervical cap is similar to the diaphragm and also must be prescribed by a doctor. It is smaller than the diaphragm, stays in place through suction, and can protect against pregnancy for up to 48 hours. The effectiveness rate of the cervical cap is about 82%, but rate can increase up to 94% if used consistently and correctly.

## Spermicidal Methods

- Vaginal Spermicides:

Vaginal spermicides are substances which are placed in the vagina and usually use nonoxynol-9 to kill sperm. They come in the form of a gel, foam, cream, or suppositories. Spermicides have a low effectiveness rate of about 79%. With correct and consistent use, however, their rate can increase to as high as 97%. The side effects may include skin irritation or a burning sensation. Spermicides are available in most drugstores.

- The Contraceptive Sponge:

The contraceptive sponge is a soft, round flexible material containing spermicide and is placed in the vagina before intercourse. The sponge provides protection for 24 hours. Its effectiveness rate is about 82%. With correct and consistent use its effectiveness rate can be as high as 94%. The sponge should not be left in place for more than 30 hours due to the possibility of toxic shock syndrome. Some women also experience vaginal dryness, difficulty removing the sponge, and a higher possibility of developing vaginal yeast infections.

## *The Least Effective Birth Control Methods*

- Withdrawal:

The withdrawal method is the removal of the penis from the vagina before ejaculation occurs. This method as a birth control has about a 82% effectiveness rate. This is because sperm may be present in the seminal fluid released by the penis just prior to ejaculation. It is also not an effective method against STDs.

- Natural Family Planning/Rhythm Method:

Many female teens believe that certain times of the month are "safe" to have intercourse because they think they "know their cycles." There are ways of determining when a woman is ovulating but these require knowledge, skill, and patience. It is best to assume that there is no safe time to have intercourse without the possibility of pregnancy. The effectiveness rate is about 80%. Using the rhythm method is also unwise because it cannot prevent the transmission of STDs.

It is important to inform teens that no physical protection can protect them from the emotional, mental, or spiritual consequences of premarital sex.

As you engage in conversation with your teen concerning sex education issues, you will see how open or closed he/she is. Your teen's openness and receptivity have a lot to do with the kind of relationship you have with him/her. Having a good relationship with your teen is absolutely essential for successful communication. These observations will help you to make practical sense of your conversations with your teen.

- Do you believe that your teen has a healthy view of his sexuality?
  Yes / No / I don't know

- Have you and your spouse already discussed reproduction with your teen?
  Yes / No / I don't know

- If the answer is Yes, how many discussions have you had?
  One        At least two        More than five

- In relation to the issues of reproduction and sexuality, how do you believe that the atmosphere in your home is best described?
  Uncomfortable        O.K., but we don't bring it up        Talk openly and freely

- If your teen came to you and wanted to know more about contraceptives, how would you feel?
  Uncomfortable/unprepared        Worried that he/she needed some        Comfortable/prepared

- After reading this section, would you like to talk to someone about these issues? Yes / No / Maybe

- If so, with whom do you plan to make an appointment?

  _____

  _____


Do the following evaluation after you have made your observations.

- How satisfied are you with your connection with your teen concerning this subject?
  Not at all satisfied        Somewhat satisfied        Very satisfied

- What have you learned about your teen's perspective of her sexuality that you did not know before this connection?

- What did you learn about yourself as a result of this connection?

- What did you learn about your spouse's perspective on sexual issues?

- Record any further insights, questions, or comments here:

## Further Resources

*None of These Diseases*, S.I. McMillen (Fleming H. Revell, division of Baker Book House, 1984).

*Talking with Your Kids about the Birds and the Bees*, Scott Talley, (Ventura: Regal Books, a division of Gospel Light Publications, 1990).

Preparing for Adolescence, Dr. James Dobson. (Ventura: Regal Books, a division of Gospel Light, 1989).

# MENTAL HEALTH

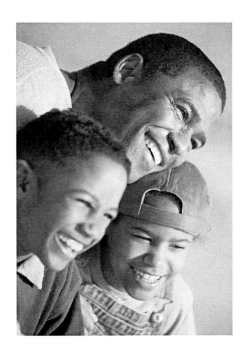

*Keep your mind active with learning new things, as well as personal and vocational development. When your mind goes into neutral, the thought life begins to crumble and questionable amusements begin to take over. Your mind is never empty. The only question is what fills it.[32]*

# C H A P T E R   N I N E

# Managing Stress

*With every passing year, we obtain a wider comprehension of the ability of the mind (psyche) to produce varied disturbances in the body (soma): hence the term psychosomatic. Invisible emotional tension in the mind can produce striking visible changes in the body, changes that can [even] become serious and fatal.*[33]

Research shows that the condition of our mental health has a profound effect upon our physical condition. Our mental health, therefore, should not be overlooked in the diagnosis of any sickness in our lives. According to Webster, a person's mental state relates to "the total emotional and intellectual response of an individual to his environment."

How can you tell if your teen is emotionally and mentally healthy? Does it mean that he must always act "happy" or "smart?" Some say that having good mental health is accepting yourself just the way you are, taking charge of your life, accepting criticism, or being able to express your thoughts and feelings freely. No matter how you try to define good mental health, it is difficult to place one specific definition on it. An important key in evaluating your teen's ability to handle stress is to ask yourself: "How well does my teen relate to his various environments?" A teen's various environments could include: home, school, youth group, church, extended family, neighborhood, team(s), and peers. It's possible for your teen to feel anxiety from any person, issue, circumstance, place, activity, or relationship in any one or more of his environments.

It's unrealistic to assume that your teen will never have to face any problems or conflicts. With the problems and conflicts, however, the Bible reminds him that there's much moral and spiritual profit to be gained:

> "...count it all joy when you fall into various trials, knowing that the testing of your faith produces patience... let patience have its perfect work, that you may be perfect and complete, lacking nothing." (James 1:2–4)

One of our major goals as parents is to help our teens understand that their happiness is a by-product of them responding to life from God's perspective. Circumstances do not have to determine their happiness. It is determined, rather, by their inner attitude or mental response to what's happening on the outside.

## 1 Know the Causes and Observe Your Teen

Stress is natural and unavoidable. A certain amount of stress is needed in order for our bodies to function. But stress is difficult to measure. One medical center describes stress as an "elusive monster, yet not an untamable one." The reason that stress is so elusive is because it is not always caused by one measurable, external event. Dr. Paul J. Rosch, clinical professor of medicine and psychiatry and president of American Institute of Stress, states: "Stress has to do with an individual's perception of ...[an] event; and, because stress is different for everyone, there is no stress-reduction regimen that works for *everyone*."

People respond differently to the same stressors. The following are some factors that affect a person's reaction to different stressors. Think of your teen when referring to the following:

- the person's age, social status, income, cultural background, stage in life, and previous experiences;

- all of the circumstances surrounding — and behind — the situation;

- how much control, or loss of control, the person has or thinks he has over the situation;

- the individual's personal relationship with God; their emotional and spiritual maturity;

- the personality of the person. Does he have a type A or type B personality?

## Is Your Teen a "Type A" or a "Type B" Person?

**Type A Characteristics:** Characteristics of a Type A personality are indicated below by any "Yes" responses.

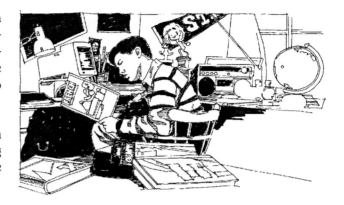

- Does your teen have a habit of explosively accentuating words in ordinary speech when there really is no need to do so? Yes / No / I don't know

- Do you notice your teen walking and/or eating rapidly even when there is no need to hurry?
  Yes / No / I don't know

- Do you notice your teen being impatient with others when she could do or say things much more quickly? Yes / No / I don't know

- Does your teen seem to feel guilty when she relaxes and does nothing for several hours? Yes / No / I don't know

- Does your teen seem to over-schedule himself and find it difficult to cut back on activities and/or responsibilities? Yes / No / I don't know

- Does your teen seem extremely agitated when he has to wait in line at a store or wait to be seated at a restaurant? Yes / No / I don't know

- Is your teen extremely competitive? Yes / No / I don't know

- Does your teen frequently try to do two or more things at once?
  Yes / No / I don't know

**Type B Characteristics:** Characteristics of a Type B personality are indicated below by any "Yes" responses.

- Does your teen seem relatively free of the traits and habits of a Type A personality as described above? Yes / No / I don't know

- Is your teen very "laid-back" and free from a sense of urgency and impatience with most anything? Yes / No / I don't know

- Is your teen more of a "back seat" listener who does not need to be the center of attention or the leader of the conversation?
Yes / No / I don't know

- Does your teen find it easy to have fun and relax? Yes / No / I don't know

- Can your teen have fun without experiencing guilt? Yes / No / I don't know

- Can your teen work without feeling agitation? Yes / No / I don't know

The more you answered "Yes" to the questions of the Type A personality, the more your teen will tend to be a Type A personality. The same applies to the Type B category of questions. If your teen has more of a Type A character, he will react differently to stress than a teen who shows more of a tendency to be a Type B. Generally, an A personality is more focused, competitive, goal-oriented, and intense than a B personality. Type A feels stress more acutely. However, most of us are a combination of both the Type A and the Type B traits. Because of their emotional intensity, parents of a Type A teen will want to make their teen aware of the increased health risks that accompany this behavior. A Type A person can learn to change the habit of always being rushed. They can learn how to live with unfinished tasks, take time to relax, and learn how to cope with daily stress in a more positive way. You can help your teen recognize this tendency and help him form a proper perspective when under stress.

If one or both parents have the tendency to exhibit Type A traits, it will be more difficult to help their teen handle his stress. The feeling of intensity in a home affects all of the children no matter what their ages. Children are very sensitive to a goal-oriented, work/duty-centered, or pressurized atmosphere.

There are both positive and negative types of stress. Positive stress causes a person to be challenged enough to face daily responsibilities and pursue goals. If there were no stressors in the life of teenagers — if they did not feel any pressure, for instance, to get out of bed to make it to school on time — their natural tendency would be to do "whatever they felt like doing." The stress of homework and chore deadlines helps teens to manage their time to feel a sense of accomplishment, and to prepare for the adult world.

There is a time, however, when positive stress can turn to negative stress. "Distress" occurs when stress reaches the point where the feelings of depression, confusion, or exhaustion replace the natural excitement and drive to meet a challenge. Instead of motivating teens to accomplish tasks, distress holds them back. The consequences of distress can be very unhealthy. Consider the following effects of negative stress. Is your teen experiencing any of these?

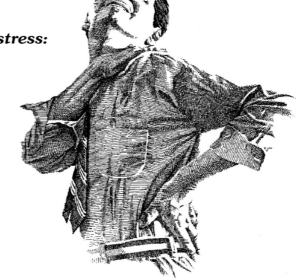

## *Physical Consequences of Distress:*

- loss of appetite
- high blood pressure
- headaches
- anorexia nervosa
- loss of menstruation
- obesity
- mononucleosis
- strep throat (repeated bouts)
- asthma
- insomnia
- extreme fatigue

## *Mental Consequences of Distress:*

- irritability
- low self-esteem
- depression
- lack of creativity
- hyper-criticalness of self and others
- low academic performance

### Social Consequences of Distress:

- uninvolved with friends
- angry outbursts
- poor time management
- lack of communication with peers and/or adults

### Spiritual Consequences of Distress:

- uninvolved in spiritual activities (youth group, etc.)
- no time to pray or read the Bible
- feelings of guilt and depression
- dissatisfaction with life
- lack of joy and purpose

## 2 Talk with Your Teen

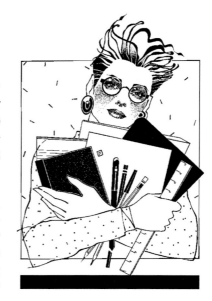

Stressors can take the form of activities, people, places, or objects. Think for a moment about your teen. Do you think he is experiencing positive or negative stress? The following section will help you determine what stress level your teen is under and give you practical ways to help your teen cope with stress.

Like other sections in *The Parent Connection*, the Conversation Starters are used to help teenagers recognize that they have a problem. After they recognize that they have a problem, they then must have a desire to do something about it. If your teen recognizes that he has a particular problem and is willing to work on solving it, then you can skip the following Conversation Starters and go directly to the Action Steps. After reading all of the following questions, choose which ones would be the most effective ways for you to use to begin a casual conversation with your teen. Remember that your purpose is to get your teen to open up — not shut down as a result of you dominating the conversation.

- *"What aspects of school are the most stressful to you? Why? How do you handle these stresses?"*

- *"What aspects of home life are the most stressful to you? Why? How do you handle these stresses?"*

- *"Did you know that there are two types of stress: positive and negative? Why do you think that doctors say that it's important to have some stress in life?"*

- *"When do you think these stresses become negative stress rather than positive stress?"*

- *"Would you say that you are experiencing positive or negative stress at this time? If it's negative stress, can you remember when the stress became negative?"*

- *"On a scale of 1 to 10, how would you rate your present ability to handle stress?" (1 = not successfully; 10 = very successfully)*

- *"On a scale of 1 to 10, how would you rate each of your family member's ability to handle stress? (1 = not successfully; 10 = very successfully) Why would you give each one the rating you did?"*

- *"Have you ever noticed what makes one stressor to you easier to deal with than another stressor?"*

- *"As an adult, how would you want to handle stress? Would you want to handle it differently than you do right now? Would you want to handle it differently than you see your mother or father handling it?"*

- *"What adult do you think copes with stress very well? Why did you choose him/her?"*

## 3 Take Action

When making observations concerning your teen's stress level, it's easy to want to relieve his stress altogether. I remember my Mother staying up late at night with me, helping me to get my assignments finished on time. She was trying to relieve the stress that I was experiencing, but it was my own procrastination that caused it. Because of my Mother's willingness to help me — and because she always had great ideas, too — I became very dependent upon her input throughout my pre-college years. In some ways her helping me only postponed the inevitable; I learned very quickly in college that Mom was not there!

Let's walk through some coping strategies that might strengthen your teen in an area where he/she does not cope well.

### ❏ Be Prepared:

Help your teen look ahead and anticipate problem situations which might create negative stress. This is totally different than operating from a base of anxiety and "borrowing trouble." If you can make a list ahead of time of what causes your teen stress, he will be better able to avoid or handle it, as the case may be. For example, you can begin working with your teen on some coping mechanisms that will help him to get mentally prepared before a competitive event, a large project, an unpleasant homework assignment, a test, a confrontation with a friend, or a meeting with a teacher or principal.

### ❏ Get Moving:

Some people live life by not taking any risks. Because they never try, they do not learn how to learn from their mistakes. Non-risk takers also never get to experience the great satisfaction that comes with facing challenges and trying new things. If people always sit and wait for God to do something supernatural for them, they might miss out on what God has for them. Let's teach our teens to trust God as they step out in faith and action.

### ❏ Manage Time:

Time management can be a natural tool to control the stress that is produced by "over-scheduling" our lives. Teens often want to be involved in more activities than they can handle. It's sometimes very difficult for them to cut back their involvements. On the other hand, there are those teens who have a difficulty managing their time even though they are not involved in any extra-curricular activities. To see if your teen realizes that he has trouble managing time, ask your teen the following questions:

- *"Do you have difficulty completing homework assignments on time?"*

- *"Do you have trouble getting to school, church, or activities on time?"*

- *"Do you feel frustrated by the lack of time you have to accomplish the things you need to do?"*

- *"Do you often feel tired and sluggish because you don't get enough sleep?"*

❏ **Get Some Exercise:**

According to fitness experts, some form of exercise three times a week is enough to help combat the effects of negative stress. Burning up that excess stress will help your teen physically and mentally cope with life's responsibilities.

❏ **Write It Down:**

Your teen is learning the benefits of journaling in the *Total Health* curriculum. When your teen records both the good and the bad of each day, it can bring him great stress-relief. Your teen can even add scriptures and/or prayers to the journal. If your teen is keeping a journal, respect his privacy and allow it to be something that no one else reads without permission. If you are concerned about what your teen might be recording in his journal, try to engage in conversations that will open him up about its contents rather than reading it without his permission.

❏ **Check Their Attitude:**

Natural coping skills are important for dealing with stress, but sometimes the attitude can play a significant part in how the stress is handled. Some call it "the principle of positive replacement" or "having a positive attitude." Whatever the case, the way we think does effect our perception of a situation. Wendell Smith, pastor of The City Church, Bellevue, Washington, teaches young people that God places a great deal of emphasis on our attitude. "We see that the emphasis that Jesus was placing in much of his teaching was not on our actions as much as it was on our attitude... our attitude determines our action."[34]

❏ **Call Regular Family Meetings:**

If a family gets into the habit of having family meetings where each person gets a time to share his thoughts and receive input and comfort from the other family members, then healthy communication can begin. Two-way communication makes teens feel that what they are going through is real, valid, and worthy of discussion.

❏ **Other Ways To Cope With Stress:**

- eat well
- get plenty of sleep
- laugh it off (have a good sense of humor!)
- talk things out with someone
- learn to relax
- set priorities
- don't let worry drain you
- learn not to procrastinate by setting small goals

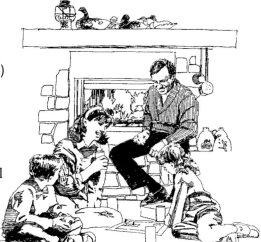

❏ **Develop An Attitude of Faith:**

Jesus talks about the power of the tongue. Our words can be a positive or negative influence in our circumstances. David, who wrote most of the Psalms, approached God in an honest yet optimistic way. He was totally honest with the Lord concerning his fears, emotions, temptations, and feelings; yet he ended his prayers with a positive confession of faith, believing that God would deliver him. We can be either an optimist or a pessimist in our approach to circumstances.

- **Optimist:** One who has the tendency to look on the more favorable side of happenings. One who minimizes adverse aspects, conditions, and possibilities, or anticipates the best possible outcome. One who sees the worst but in complete realism, still believing in the best. One who has a cheerful or hopeful temperament.

- **Pessimist:** One who has the tendency to see what is gloomy or anticipate the worst possible outcome.

An attitude of faith in God's sovereignty is what will determine much of a person's ability to handle negative stress. Parents of teens who are experiencing stress, can help them cope by speaking faith and encouraging them to look to God as their source of peace and strength.

> "You will keep him in perfect peace, whose mind is stayed on You, because he trusts in You." Isaiah 26:3

❏ After going through this section, what do you feel your teen is experiencing?

No stress          A healthy amount of stress          Negative stress          Extreme stress

❏ List below the ways that you and your family can help your teen handle stress better:

_____

_____

_____

_____

## 4 Pause to Reflect

After you finish the appropriate Action Steps, complete this evaluation to see how the chapter worked for you.

● How well did you "connect" with your teen through this material?

Not very well          Fairly well          Very well

● What did you learn about your teen and his/her ability to handle stress?




● What did you learn about the way you handle stress?




● How successful were the Conversation Starters with your teen?

Not successful                    Somewhat successful                    Very successful

- Record any further insights, questions, or comments concerning your teen and stress here:

## Further Resources

*Balancing Life's Demands*, A New Perspective on Priorities, J. Grant Howard, Multnomah Press, 1983.

*The Relaxed Parent.* Helping Your Kids Do More as You Do Less, Tim Smith, Northfield Publishing, 1996.

*Pressures, Finding the Balance, Seven Lessons on Lifestyle,* Lyman Coleman, Serendipity House, 1994.

*The Hidden Link Between Adrenaline and Stress,* Dr. Archibald D. Hart, Word Publishing, 1995.

# CHAPTER TEN

# Depression

*Life was given you by God… in a great big box with a wonderful ribbon on it… what we expect in there is joy, peace, contentment, and an abundance of love. But we also find in that life, pain, despair and loneliness. They are all part of the same box called life. It's not until you dive into it and experience all of it that you will really know life. We learn from pain just as much as we learn from joy.*[35]

Life is filled will situations that cause stress. If we examine the life of an adult and compare it to the life of a teenager, we find many of the same conflicts. Adults worry about their appearance and social acceptance. They experience problems with peer pressure, and have conflicts at work and at home. What we often overlook is that teens face difficult challenges but do not have the perspective or emotional maturity that can help them go through them positively. Many teens feel they are dealing with their problems alone. When teens go to their peers for counsel and support, they gain the same immature perspective that may only reinforce their feeling of depression.

Mike Miller, a national speaker and founder of Dare To Live, compares depression to the common cold. It's like the common cold of mental disorders:

> "It starts with the sniffles; no one dies of the sniffles. But without proper care, a cold (or depression) can progress from the sniffles to a head cold, to a chest cold and even to pneumonia… plenty of people die from pneumonia."[36]

## 1 Know the Causes and Observe Your Teen

If you were to ask several teenagers if they have ever been depressed, the answer would be a unanimous "yes." Times of depression are common for both teenagers as well as adults. That "sad and blue" feeling, that overwhelming feeling of hopelessness and worthlessness, that feeling of disappointment, can lead to apathy and withdrawal.

The following is a list of a few general reasons why teenagers may experience depression:

- A teenager's changing hormones and unstable emotional state.

- A symptom that shows that something is not right or needs to be worked through.

- A response to stress and life events: academics, arguments with friends and family, a move of family or friend, a loss of a loved one or conflicts at home.

- A reaction to feelings of guilt, bitterness, unresolved anger or unresolved grief.

- A response to the high expectations of others and the pressure to succeed.

- A lack of the revelation of the unconditional love of God. Usually associated with the feelings that "I'm not good enough."

Whatever way you describe depression, the disorder can range from occasional to extreme. Experiencing some depression is normal for everyone. However, if you feel your teen shows signs of prolonged depression it might be signs of a more serious problem. For most teens, the feeling of depression will lift after a short period of time. In more serious circumstances, teenagers need to find someone with whom they can share their feelings.

As you make the following observations concerning your teenager, try to look beyond these signs of depression to see if you can find a deeper cause to his/her behavior.

- Does your teen have a difficult time sleeping at night? Yes / No / I don't know

- Has your teen's appetite decreased? Yes / No / I don't know

- Does your teen seem bored and unmotivated lately? Yes / No / I don't know

- Has your teen lost interest in activities that used to interest him/her?
  Yes / No / I don't know

- Does your teen seem distracted and unable to concentrate? Yes / No / I don't know

- Has your teen complained about feeling more tired lately? Yes / No / I don't know

- Does your teen just not get out of bed in the morning? Yes / No / I don't know

- Has your teen not been as talkative as he/she usually is? Yes / No / I don't know

- Does your teen have a preoccupation with death, dying, or suicide?
  Yes / No / I don't know

- Has your teen been severely depressed for more than one week?
  Yes / No / I don't know

- Has your teen made any off-handed remarks such as, "You won't be seeing me much longer" or, "If anything should happen to me?" Yes / No / I don't know

- Does your teen show signs of low self-esteem, feelings of worthlessness, or self-hatred? Yes / No / I don't know

If you answered Yes to six or more of the Observation questions, your teen may be experiencing deep depression. The last four questions are warning signs of suicide. This observation section is not intended to alarm you. It is meant to help you notice a significant change in behavior or attitude and then take any practical steps to help your teen overcome the deepening depression.

## 2 Talk with Your Teen

If you cannot determine any specific reason why your teen may be depressed, you may want to use the following Conversation Starters to help open up communication. Depression usually leads to withdrawal and an "I don't care" attitude. The sooner you open up conversation, the less likely the depression will escalate.

In the United States alone, an estimated one million people a year try to take their own lives. Suicide is the second leading cause of death among adolescents with fatalities of more than 6,000 a year (the first is accidents). Why do so many young people try to commit suicide? The answer varies with each individual. However, an overwhelming feeling of worthlessness and hopelessness is an underlying factor. In one study, when those who had survived a suicide attempt were asked why they tried to take their lives, the majority answered, "because nobody cares."

"Very few people who attempt suicide really want to die, the overwhelming majority of those who are lucky enough to be helped... never try suicide again."[37]

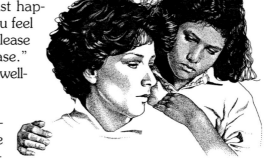

Good communication between parent(s) and their teenager(s) is a process and will not just happen with one or two conversations. If you feel that your teen will not respond to you, please don't give up or leave it as "just a phase." People who are trained in counseling are well-equipped to help your teen.

After reading all of the following questions, choose which ones would be the most effective ways for you to use to begin a casual conversation with your teen. Remember that your purpose is to get your teen to open up — not shut down as a result of you dominating the conversation.

- *"Do you think adults get depressed?"*

- *"What do you think adults get depressed about?"*

- *"What do you think teens get depressed about?"*

- *"When you feel depressed, how do you feel?"*

- *"What causes you to feel depressed the most often?"*

- *"If you could change anything in your life, what would you change? Why?"*

- *"If you lived on a desert island, with whom would you like to live?"*

- *"If you could go to heaven right now and ask God anything, what would you ask Him?"*

- *"If you knew of a friend who was talking about taking his life, what would you say to him?"*

- *"How do you think God feels about a person who wants to take his life?"*

- *"How can a person's faith in God help when the feeling of depression is so deep?"*

## 3 Take Action

When trying to communicate with your teen about deep, emotional issues, it can seem very overwhelming. Maybe she opens up right away, you have a great conversation, and the problem gets resolved. Unfortunately, this is not usually the case. Most of the time, teens have a difficult time sharing their deep thoughts and feelings. They may feel you will make light of their feelings with a response such as: "I don't see why you'd feel that way at all, you'll get over it in time." Teens may feel embarrassed to share with you some deep emotional hurts that they have felt for a long time. Very often, teens who are experiencing depression do not have the words to describe a specific situation that is causing these feelings. Whatever your teen's situation, validate her feelings by acknowledging the situation through acceptance, love, comfort, and affection.

❏ After reading this section and observing your teen, do you feel your teen has a problem with depression? Yes / No / I don't know

❏ What seems to be the main reason for your teen's depression?


❏ Do you feel that your teen has thoughts of suicide? Yes / No / I don't know

❏ If you think you have reason to be concerned, list the appropriate people to contact, along with their telephone numbers, below:

- A trusted teacher at school:_____

  _____

- A close friend:_____

  _____

- A youth pastor/leader at church:_____

_____

- A trusted school counselor:_____

_____

- Other siblings in the family who are old enough to understand:_____

_____

❑ Talk to your spouse in detail about your concerns and have your spouse share his/her insights.

❑ If you feel there's a reason to be concerned, address your teen about his behavior and attitude and encourage him to talk to someone about it. Most probably, you should go with your teen if he chooses to talk to an adult other than yourself or your spouse.

❑ List several practical ways that you'll make an effort to be involved in your teen's life.

- _____

- _____

- _____

❑ Make an effort to spend time with your teen alone doing something he really likes to do.

❑ Make a special effort to pray for your teen daily and ask the Lord for wisdom concerning his situation.

# 4 **Pause to Reflect**

After you finish the appropriate Action Steps, complete this evaluation to see how the chapter worked for you.

- How well did you "connect" with your teen in this section?

  Not very well          Fairly well          Very well

- What did you learn about your teen that you did not know before?


- What did you learn about your family as a result of this material?


- What did you learn about yourself as a result of this chapter?


- How successful were the Conversation Starters with your teen?

  Not successful          Somewhat successful          Very successful

- How successful were the Action Steps in your situation?

  Not successful   Somewhat successful Very successful

- Record any further insights, questions, or comments concerning depression and your teen here:

# Further Resources

*Where is God When It Hurts,* Philip Yancey, Zondervan Publishing, 1977.

*Helping The Struggling Adolescent: A Guide to 30 Common Problems for Parents, Counselors, and Youth Workers,* Les Parrott III, Zondervan, 1993.

*Preparing For Adolescence,* Dr. James Dobson, Regal Books, 1978.

*Habits of the Mind, Ten Exercises to Renew Your Thinking,* Dr. Archibald D. Hart, Word Publishing, 1996.

*Suicide Survivors: A Guide for those Left Behind,* Adina Wrobleski, Afterwords Publishing, 1994.

*Suicide: Why? 85 Questions and Answers About Suicide,* Adina Wrobleski, Afterwords Publishing, 1995.

*Grief: Dying, Death & Destiny,* Herbert Lockyer, Revell, Baker Book House, 1980.

*Counsel Yourself and Others From the Bible,* Bob Moorehead, Multnomah Press, 1994.

# Developing the Three C's:
## Conduct, Character, Conviction

*And do not be conformed to this world, but be transformed by the renewing of your mind, that you may prove what is that good and acceptable and perfect will of God. (Romans 12:2)*

No matter what religion or nationality, it's every parent's goal that their child matures into a responsible adult. This means that his lifestyle (whole way of living) will be acceptable to God and responsible to others. For Christians, a person's lifestyle incorporates a different standard than what might be acceptable in society. As a result, parents of teenagers are challenged to teach their teens to avoid conformity with the world and not to be afraid to stand-out-of-the-crowd.

In this section of *The Parent Connection*, we're going to concentrate on the lifestyle of a teen. When the word lifestyle is mentioned, it's often associated with a person's financial stability. However, people's lifestyles are not only measured by how they may live financially, but more importantly, they're measured by their conduct, character, and convictions. For your teen to reach his full potential and become the best possible person he can be, your teen must learn to manage his lifestyle. Many of the decisions teens make now will have an effect upon what kind of lifestyle they will have as an adult. This not only includes the habits that are revealed in their conduct, but also the character and convictions they are building deep inside.

## 1 Know the Causes

Let's begin with some functional definitions:

- **Conduct:** I want my child to have a high, godly standard of behavior.

- **Character:** I want my child to develop the character of Christ, to have strong moral excellence and the ability to stand firm in the midst of negative pressure.

- **Conviction:** I want my child to develop personal and biblical convictions that will give structure and guidance to his life.

How and when these lifestyle ingredients develop is very individual and personal, but it's often in the teen years that parents begin to see a young adult emerge. It's this time when teens are seeking independence and gaining more responsibility. These teenagers will be young adults soon, and they will reflect the years of choices and habits that they have developed.

In order to avoid conforming to the world in his lifestyle, your teen needs to be transformed by the renewing of his mind. A teen can learn discipline not only in the practical areas of life, but can also learn to discipline his mind. A teenager's thoughts as well as actions will form habits that sooner or later will become his lifestyle. The student text explains this principle using the acronym G.I.G.O. — "Garbage In — Garbage Out" or, "Good In — Good Out."

The ability of your teen to develop godly convictions of his own will depend on how he becomes a "Wisdom Thinker." [38] Authors Carolyn Kohlenberger and Noel Wescombe in their book *Raising Wise Children*, list and explain the three skills of Wisdom Thinking:

1. Gathering, Sorting, and Choosing
2. Thinking about Thinking
3. Thinking about God

### 1. Gathering, Sorting, and Choosing:

"The first step is gathering information.... We gather information almost constantly. We hear or read a new fact or idea, and we store it away. We see a new object... we touch, smell, and taste.... We go out and gather new 'outside' information and add it to the old 'inside' information. But gathering information is not enough when deciding what to believe or do. Thinkers must learn to sort what is useful from what is not.... When we have sorted and found what options are open to us, we must then choose what we will believe or do.... Imagine [that] you own a factory where you make apple pies... You go outside to the orchard and gather as many apples as you can.... You take the apples to your factory and dump them on the conveyor belt. As it rolls by, you sort them. Some cannot be used because they're rotten or bruised, but others are just right... Then you bake all the ingredients together. Out of those finished pies, taste reveals the best pie. You choose that pie to serve to your customers." [39]

### 2. Thinking about Thinking:

Thinking about Thinking has three parts, too. "The first part is looking ahead — it is planning how to think. The second part is keeping a close eye on thinking while gathering, sorting, and choosing. The third part is looking back to see how well thinking was done....[Each of these parts will help your teen distinguish between fact and opinion.] Now go back to your apple pie factory. Thinking about Thinking takes the role of your plant manager. She checks to see that all the machinery is in working order before the conveyor belt begins to roll. [She] makes sure all the workers are in their stations. Then she carefully watches them while they work. She listens to the machines.... Thinking about Thinking protects the outcome of your thought process. Knowing where problems can pop up, and seeing to it that they don't, keeps thinking on track." [40]

### 3. Thinking about God:

Thinking about God also has three parts. "The first part is learning to use God's Word as a part of thinking, the second part is listening to wise counselors, and the third part is praying while thinking. Without the skill of Thinking about God, we are no better than human computers.... A loving, caring, and eternal perspective cannot be programmed into computers....

[In your apple pie factory,] Thinking about God oversees the work with Thinking about Thinking, though Thinking about God has more seniority. In his hands he holds the 'Recipe' for the best apple pie the world has ever tasted." [41]

So, how does the skill of thinking help a teenager in the areas of his conduct, character and conviction? Wise thinking is not only given by God's grace, but it's also a learned and practiced skill. Daily, parents can help their teens understand and practice the connection between thought patterns and eventual lifestyle.

The following questions will give you a thermometer of your teen's conduct, character, and convictions. The Action Steps will focus on what kind of convictions your teen is developing.

## 2  Observe Your Teen

## Observations of Conduct

A person's true character is displayed by what he does when no one else is watching. I recently had the opportunity to watch my son interact with a neighbor while they were playing together in the backyard. It was interesting to observe my son's behavior and listen to his conversation when he didn't know that I was watching. It's a good test for us to listen and observe our children closely. Although such observations are embarrassing at times, a good way of doing this is to ask those close to us what they see in our children when we are not present.

- Do you approve of your teen's choices in friends?

    Not at all     Some of the friends     All of the friends

- Does your teen respond to the boundaries that you set for her?

    Not at all     Sometimes     All of the time

- Are you always aware of where your teen is and who he is with when gone?

    Not at all     Sometimes     All of the time

- Do you feel that you can trust your teen when you are not around?

    Not at all     Sometimes     All of the time

- Do other parents think well of your teen? Yes / No / I don't know

- What have you heard from others concerning your teen?
  A few bad comments    Only bad comments    A few good comments    Only good comments

- Has your teen ever been in trouble with the law? Yes / No / I don't know

Conduct is a standard of personal behavior. It's what people see revealed in actions and attitudes. It takes a lifestyle of self-discipline and self-control to help develop good habits of conduct. We don't expect our teens to be perfect in every way, but if we can observe their conduct more closely it might lead us to understand what's happening on a deeper level.

## Observations of Character

How can you observe your teen's inner character? Your teen's character is comprised of his personal integrity, true motivations, daily habits, most frequent thought patterns, dominant desires, controlling values, and conscious convictions. Your teenager's inner character is revealed in his unique actions and attitudes that set him apart from others. Teens don't have to act "religious" to demonstrate true character. In fact, it's genuine love and humility that are the cornerstones of Christian character. Such love and humility was best shown to us in the life of Jesus. Jesus always put His Father's will and the other person's best interest (their highest spiritual good) first. There is no "faking" or "acting" involved in true character.

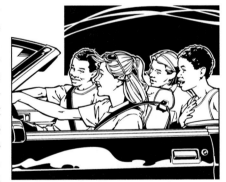

I've seen too many young people simply "play the part" of a Christian in an effort to impress their parents and/or church leaders. One common cause of such play acting (hypocrisy) is parents who emphasize to their teens an outward conformity to many religious rules and obligations rather than allowing them to develop a sincere inner relationship with the Lord at their own pace. Having character that's inherent is obviously important:

"Having character is much like having class. Class is having a standard of high quality that sets you apart from the crowd. If you do have class, you don't need much of anything else. If you don't have it, no matter what else you have, it doesn't make much difference." [42]

"How people play the game shows some of their character; how they win it or lose it shows it all."[43]

Use the following questions to help you discern your teen's inner character.

- If your teen is involved in any competitive game or event — even a board game — is she a good loser? Yes / No / Sometimes

- If your teen is involved in any competitive game or event — even a board game — is he a good winner? Yes / No / Sometimes

- Is your teen honest? Yes / No / Sometimes

- Does your teen have a clear conscience before others, i.e., no serious unresolved offenses? Yes / No / I don't know

- Do you believe that your teen is morally pure? Yes / No / I don't know

- Do you believe that your teen is forgiving and doesn't hold grudges?
  Yes / No / I don't know

- Do you believe that your teen doesn't have a problem with anger?
  Yes / No / I don't know

- Generally, does your teen put the needs of others before himself?
  Yes / No / I don't know

Character is not something that someone develops overnight or learns in a class. Godly character is facilitated by the home and deposited by God's grace into a teen's life. It takes hard work, personal experiences, counsel, learning from mistakes, and discipline over a period of time. Character is formed by *events* occurring in a teen's life. These events can be either positive or negative experiences, and the development of character depends upon the individual's responses to them. Sometimes we can be too hard on our teens expecting them to be "perfect in all their ways." God will continue to work in their lives as they give Him opportunity. Obviously, the best way that parents can facilitate the continued development of godly character in the life of their teen is through their own daily example.

## Observations of Convictions

"A conviction is a personal belief upon which certain actions are based. It is the motivation or reason behind the action… A conviction must have a base — convictions do not emerge fully formed… Developing convictions is not an event but a process. It is step-by-step unfolding — a developing process that leads to a conclusion… Convictions should be personal… and also biblical."[44]

For years you have tried to teach your child the values and beliefs that have formed your lifestyle. Nevertheless, you may still find that many of your answers to the following observations are "I don't know." That's OK. Through **The Parent Connection**, you will be getting to know your teen even more. At the end of the list, there's a space where you can add any other area of conviction. When you reflect upon your teen's personal convictions, it will be helpful to keep in mind that the same conviction can be worded either in a posi- 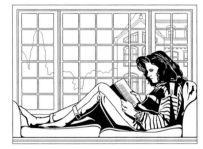 tive or negative form. E.g., a teen's conviction against abortion can be worded either: "I strongly believe in the right of the unborn" or, "I'm strongly opposed to the pro-choice position." Either way, the statement describes the same conviction.

The following questions will help you to begin to identify your own teen's set of personal convictions up to this point in his life:

- Does your teen have a conviction against lying? Yes / No / I don't know

- Does your teen have a conviction against stealing?
  Yes / No / I don't know

- Does your teen have a conviction which opposes cheating?
  Yes / No / I don't know

- Does your teen have a conviction about sexual standards?
  Yes / No / I don't know

- Does your teen have a conviction concerning respecting authority?

  Yes / No / I don't know

- Does your teen have a conviction about television viewing or music listening?

  Yes / No / I don't know

- Does your teen have a conviction about the literature she reads?

  Yes / No / I don't know

- Does your teen have a conviction about the videos or movies he watches?

  Yes / No / I don't know

- Does your teen have a conviction about prayer? Yes / No / I don't know

- Does your teen have a conviction about the Bible and Bible reading?

  Yes / No / I don't know

- If your teen has a strong conviction not mentioned in the above list, or, if you would like to ask her about a certain area, record it here:

It's often difficult for parents to know for sure what their teens really believe. Teenagers may not know how strongly they feel about an issue until their conviction is tested. Unfortunately for young people, one of the ways that their convictions are tested is through temptations. It's important to use **The Parent Connection** to help your teen(s) to develop strong personal standards before they are faced with compromising situations. Does your teen have strong convictions? Does your teen have the fortitude to stand by these convictions in the face of peer opposition? Does your teen have the courage to be different? Are their convictions their own?

## Helping Teens Develop Their Own Convictions

After honestly asking your teen to answer the questions concerning his conduct, character, and convictions, you may feel unsure about whether or not your teen is developing the lifestyle that will make him into a responsible Christian adult. The following steps will help you to guide your teen in the formation of convictions that he can call his own.

Even some parents do not always know what they believe or why they believe it. Teens are going through so many changes that their actions may seem to be contrary to some of the strong beliefs that their parents have been working so hard to instill in them. Developing strong, personal convictions is a process. To encourage the conviction formation process, parents can use the following questions with their teen(s):

### Developing Convictions

Does it glorify God? (I Corinthians 10:31; Philippians 1:20)

What does the Bible say about the issue? (John 14:21; I Samuel 15:22)

Is it helpful to you physically, mentally, and spiritually? (I Corinthians 6:12; Philippians 4:8)

Does it enslave you and bring you under its power? (I Corinthians 6:12)

Does it hurt others or cause others to stumble in their faith? (I Corinthians 8: 9,13; Hebrews 10:24)

Developing biblical convictions in your teen is only the first step in the process of Christian maturity. An equally important question is, "Will my teen live by his convictions?" To begin a dialogue with your teen about this, you can use the following Conversation Starters.

## 3 Talk with Your Teen

After reading all of the following questions, choose which ones would be the most effective ways for you to use to begin a casual conversation with your teen. Remember that your purpose is to get your teen to open up — not shut down as a result of you dominating the conversation.

- *"What do you think it means to have a conviction about something?"*

- *"What convictions or strong beliefs have you seen in our family?"*

- *"Of these strong beliefs, which ones do you agree with and which ones do you not agree with?"*

- *"What convictions will you try to teach to your children?"*

- *"What convictions will you teach differently to your children?"*

- *"If a friend of yours was caught cheating at school, how would you feel toward your friend? Would you say anything to your friend? If so, what?"*

- *"If your best friend wanted you to go with him to see a movie that your parent's did not want you to see, what would you do?"*

- *"If a close friend wanted you to lie about where you were going to go, what would you do?"*

- *"If your best friend told you that he was sleeping with the person he was dating, how would you feel about your friend? Would you tell your friend that you disagreed with what he was doing? Would you continue being his best friend even though he did not change his behavior?"*

- *"If the Bible did not say anything specific about a certain issue, how would you go about developing an opinion or conviction about it?"*

## 4 Take Action

When assisting your teen in the development of personal — yet biblical — convictions, it's difficult many times for a parent to remember that God has given everyone a free will. Our teens will disappoint us. They will even disagree with our standards. However, through prayer, an open relationship with Mom and Dad, persistent love, and unending patience, parents can have the confidence that their children will avoid major compromises and fulfill God's will for their lives.

Consider the following Action Steps to help you to continue what you have already started with your teen.

❏ After reading this section and observing your teen, which of the following best describes your teen's conduct?

    Below what I expected      In line with what I expected      Above what I expected

❏ In what area does your teen have the most difficulty developing a strong, biblical conviction?



❏ Do you feel that your teen is truly sincere about his religious convictions, or do you think that he is mostly putting on a good act to impress others or keep the pressure off?

❏ After reading this section, and observing and talking with your teen, which of the following best describes your teen's present conviction level?

    Below what I expected      In line with what I expected      Above what I expected

❏ Do you feel that your teen is withholding any important information from you perhaps because he does not want to disappoint you, or fears that you will become extremely angry?

❏ After reading this section and observing your teen, which of the following best describes your teen's inner character?

    Below what I expected      In line with what I expected      Above what I expected

❏ Talk with one of your teen's friend's parent(s) concerning how they perceive your teen. (This needs to be a trustworthy friend who can honestly evaluate your teen; also, someone at whose comments you will not be offended.)

❏ Speak to your teen's youth leader at church. Ask him/her for any input about your son or daughter.

❏ Discuss your teen's conduct, character, and convictions with your spouse in private. Share in-depth and pray with each other about the weak areas of your teen's life.

❏ Pray more often for your teen. Pray that he will become increasingly sensitive to the moving of the Holy Spirit in his life and to the development of biblical convictions.

## *5* Pause to Reflect

After you finish the appropriate Action Steps, complete this evaluation to see how the chapter worked for you.

• How well did you "connect" with your teen in this section?

Not very well                 Fairly well                 Very well

• What did you learn about your teen's convictions that you didn't know before this section?


• What did you learn about your family's convictions as a result of this chapter?


• What did you learn about your own convictions as a result of this information?


• How successful were the Action Steps in your situation?

Not successful            Somewhat successful            Very successful

• How successful were the Conversation Starters with your teen?

Not successful            Somewhat successful            Very successful

• Record any further insights, questions, or comments concerning this section and your teen here:

## Further Resources

*Honesty, Morality and Conscience,* Jerry White, Navpress, 1983.

*Right from Wrong,* Josh McDowell and Bob Hostetler, Word Publishing, 1994.

*Raising Kids Who Turn Out Right,* Tim Kimmel, Multnomah Press, 1989.

*The Teen's Topical Bible, Real Answers for the Problems only Teens Face,* The Living Bible, Honor Books.

*The Walk, The Measure of Spiritual Maturity*, Gene A. Getz, Broadman & Holman Publishing, 1994.

*Victory, The Principles of Championship Living,* A.C. Green, Creation House, 1994.

# Friendships and Peer Pressure

A study conducted by NFO Research, Inc., found the following influences to be the most significant, according to the teenagers polled:

### According to Teenagers, What's the Single Worst Influence Facing Teens Today?

You and your family may live in an area where drug use is more prevalent or

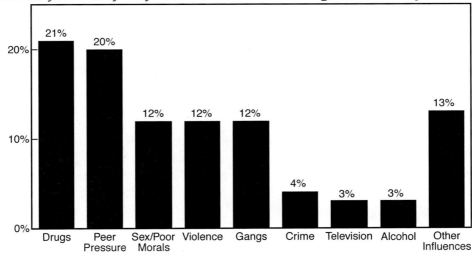

less prevalent than other families, however, the influence of peer pressure runs a close second to drugs as the worst influence facing teens. It's interesting to note that these are the influences that the teenagers themselves picked — not adults projecting their own personal opinions onto the situation. Do you think teenagers realize how much their peers influence their decisions? Personally, I do. However, I don't believe that teenagers realize how negative the influence is.

"The influence of people on people is a powerful force, affecting everyone. Only the power of God and the innate drive for physical survival outrank it. A reasoning mind can become powerless in the face of this pressure. Even the most committed individualist conforms in some ways to the lifestyle of others." [45]

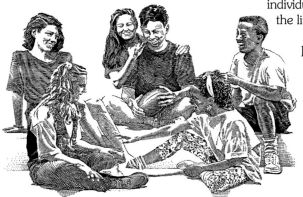

I remember being a teenager and thinking, "I must be going crazy!" There were so many thoughts and feelings going on inside of me that I didn't know what to do. My moods were in a constant state of change. Any little aggravation from my environment set me off. The increased pressures in society have caused teens more confusion. Decisions aren't as clear as they once were, and the matter of right and wrong is often confusing. In short, teenagers have much more to "think about" and "sort through."

The pressures that teens feel, however, can easily get exaggerated as a result of the many physical changes happening in their bodies. These changes will directly affect a teen's thoughts. Teenagers will have thoughts about the opposite sex that they have not had before. Some teens may even have thoughts about having romantic/sexual friendships with members of the same sex. Especially in today's society, such thoughts may encourage them to believe that they are homosexual. Teens will have all kinds of thoughts. These many ideas that pass through their minds are normal. Most of them are due simply to unstable hormones. The hormones causing a teen's body to change can also be responsible for feelings of frustration, fear, inadequacy, and depression — at home or at school. It's vital that *every* teen finds a responsible Christian adult to talk to about their feelings.

The influence of a non-Christian culture on a teen's mind may be very subtle, but the fear of being different is a very strong emotion. The temptation to conform to the group can keep Christian young people from doing what is right. Every teen is tempted to conform to his peers in speech, behavior, and eventually lifestyle.

In our society, the ethical and moral standards of former days are virtually non-existent. The prevalent ethic in America today is one of total self-interest: do whatever feels good at the moment — just make sure you don't get caught. Self-interest affects people of all ages. It's obvious that teens will not become morally strong as a result of a single discussion with their parents about making wise choices. Moral development is a process that parents work hard at all their child's life. It seems as though the adolescent years are the testing ground. Let's look at some concrete ideas that parents can do to help their teens avoid falling into the trap of peer pressure.

## *1*  Know the Causes

Why are some teens less affected by peer pressure than others? The following is a list of some of the factors that contribute to a teenager's ability to avoid conformity:

- The stability of the teenager's home life

- The level of the teenager's self-esteem

- The amount of positive feedback the teenager receives from significant others

- The physical health of the teenager

- The sense of destiny or purpose that the teenager feels

- The depth of the teenager's relationship with God

- The friends with whom the teenager associates

- The in-born personality of the teenager (is he/she a follower or a leader?)

- The strength of the teenager's personal convictions

Turn your attention to your own teen. Answer the following questions as you try to determine how your teen is handling the temptation to conform to peer pressure.

## 2 Observe Your Teen

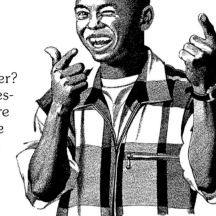

- Is your teen more naturally a leader?

  Yes / No / I don't know

- Is your teen more naturally a follower? (Being more of a follower is not necessarily wrong. We're speaking here more of a personality type and tendency. The danger for a follower, however, is if he allows himself to be led by the wrong people in the wrong direction.) Yes / No / I don't know

- When you observe your teen with his/her friends, how often do you see him/her give in to their wishes?

  Not often at all        Somewhat often        Very often

- When you observe your teen with her friends, how often do you see her friends follow her choices or ideas?

  Not often at all        Somewhat often        Very often

- Have you ever asked your teen how peer pressure makes him feel?

  Not often at all        Somewhat often        Very often

- Do you feel that your teen's friends are being a positive influence in her life?
  Yes / No / I don't know

- Do you believe that your teen has a strong feeling of purpose and destiny in his life? Yes / No / I don't know

- How strong do you believe your teen's relationship with the Lord is?

  Weak        Average        Very strong

- Do you think that your teen feels comfortable talking with you about peer pressure? Yes / No / I don't know

- How often do you think your teen's friends cause him to compromise his values?

   Neveer        Sometimes        I don't know

- Do you think your teen is a good friend and a positive influence to others?

   Yes        Sometimes        No        I don't know

- Do you think your teen fills her time wisely and stays busy with constructive activities?

   Yes        Sometimes        No        I don't know

## 3 Talk with Your Teen

It's very good when teens tell their parents about peer pressure, but it's even better when they tell their parents how they are responding to it on the inside. It's sometimes difficult to know exactly how your teen is responding to the temptation to conform; but open communication is a key. The communication between you and your teen must be a two-way dialogue. To be successful, your teen needs to feel that he can be honest with his feelings and/or failures.

After reading all of the following questions, choose which ones would be the most effective ways for you to use to begin a casual conversation with your teen. Remember that your purpose is to get your teen to open up — not shut down as a result of you dominating the conversation.

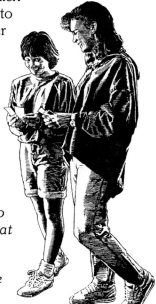

- *"What would you say is the strongest peer pressure you face?"*

- *"What do you feel is the best way you handle peer pressure?"*

- *"If you knew a friend was being pressured into doing something he/she did not want to do, what would you say to him/her?"*

- *"What do you feel is your strongest defense against peer pressure?"*

- *"Do you think there's any difference in the way an adult might handle peer pressure and the way that a teen might handle it?"*

- *"How do you see your friends handling peer pressure?"*

- *"What do you feel is the most important attribute in a friend?"*

- *"Do you have a best friend? Why is he/she your best friend?"*

- *"How can the way you think in your mind affect the way you respond in a group?"*

- *"How do you think society and the media try to influence teens? Does it work?" Explain.*

## 4 Take Action

The goal of this connection was to help you better understand what your teen is facing. It was also to give you a better insight into how your teen is responding to peer pressure. The following Action Steps will provide you with some practical ways to put this section into practice.

❏ After reading this section, do you feel that your teen has a good handle on dealing with peer pressure?

Yes     Sometimes     No
I don't know

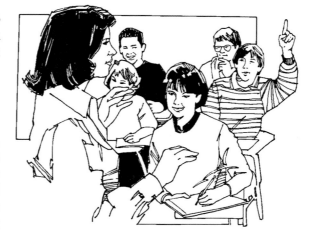

❏ After reading this section, choose several people to talk to who will be able to give you a fuller understanding of what conformity pressures your teen faces and what might be done to help him.

- _____
- _____
- _____

❏ Plan a regular "family night" or "family meeting" in which family members can openly share any frustrations caused at home or elsewhere. During these meetings, give your children your undivided attention. You might want to choose a certain subject each time to help prompt discussion. Don't get stuck on an unfruitful topic, however. Go with where the flow of the discussion is constructively going. Be careful not to make the gathering into a time of correction.

❏ What is the most difficult area that your teen deals with in terms of conformity and peer pressure?

❏ How can you help your teen grow in this area?

❏ After reading this section, do you feel that your teen has too much spare time on his hands? Encourage your teen to get involved in something that he would enjoy doing. This will help to keep your teen's mind and body active. List some ideas that you came up with together below:

● _____

● _____

● _____

❏ Pray daily that your teen will have the strength and the grace to overcome every temptation to negative peer influence. One possible prayer is: "Lord, no matter what her personality or gifting, make her a moral and spiritual leader with whomever she comes into contact."

## *5* Pause to Reflect

After you finish the appropriate Action Steps, complete this evaluation to see how the chapter worked for you.

● How well did you "connect" with your teen through this material?

Not very well        Fairly well        Very well

- What did you learn about your teen and peer pressure that you didn't know before?

- What did you learn about your family as a result of this section?

- What did you learn about yourself as a result of this chapter? (How well do you respond to adult peer pressure?)

- How successful were the Action Steps in your situation?

  Not successful          Somewhat successful          Very successful

- Record any further insights, questions, or comments concerning this section and your teen here:

## Further Resources

*Belonging: 7 Sessions on Friendships,* Lyman Coleman, Serendipity House, 1994.

*Welcome To High School,* Diane Eble, et. al., Campus Life Books, Zondervan, 1991.

*What Your Kids Are Up To And In For,* Bill Sanders, Fleming Revell, 1992.

# CHAPTER THIRTEEN

# A Teen's Emotional Earthquakes

*Young people feel more strongly about everything, especially during adolescence... Little things that won't bother you later in life will bug you as a teenager. Your fears will be more frightening, your pleasures will be more exciting, your irritations will be more distressing, and your frustrations will be more intolerable. Every experience will appear king-sized....*[46]

## 1 Know the Causes

Earthquakes occur naturally and are caused by a shifting or a change in the earth. A certain degree of trembling and shaking occur as a result. Some earthquakes cause major damage, while others cause no more than a slight disturbance. All parents of teens experience some form of an earthquake in their home at some time during the adolescent period. Generally, there are no exceptions to this. The physical changes that occur in a teen's body directly affect his thoughts, attitudes, and feelings. It's how you and your teen handle these earthquakes that will determine their ultimate result.

Many of the changes that your teen will experience are closely related to her emotions. Emotions are those often unpredictable feelings that can cause teenagers to say or do things that they later regret. All teens experience the roller-coaster ride of emotional upheaval. It's good to be aware that the most common emotions dealt with during adolescence have to do with:

- A teenager's feelings about God

- A teenager's feelings about his parents and family

- A teenager's feelings about his friends

- A teenager's feelings about his self-identity

Use the following questions as a thermometer of your teen's thoughts and feelings in these four main areas.

## 2 Observe Your Teen

### Your teen's feelings about God

- Has your teen had some Christian teaching since birth?
  Yes / No / I don't know

- Has your teen only recently had some Christian teaching (during the last four years)? Yes / No / I don't know

- Has your teen asked questions concerning God and Christianity that cause you to doubt his personal faith? Yes / No / I don't know

- Does your teen seem to enjoy going to church? Yes / No / I don't know

- Does your teen initiate conversations about God while alone with you and the family? Yes / No / I don't know

- Does your teen take the initiative to pray in groups?
  Yes / No / I don't know

### Your teen's feelings about parents and family

- Does your teen seem to enjoy going to family functions?
  Yes / No / I don't know

- Does there seem to be an obvious generation gap between you and your teen?
  Yes / No / I don't know

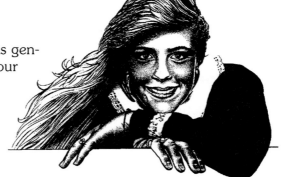

- Does there seem to be an obvious generation gap between your spouse and your teen?

  Yes / No / I don't know

- Does your teen seem to get along well with his siblings?

  Yes / No / I don't know

- Has your teen made positive remarks concerning marriage and family living?

  Yes / No / I don't know

### Your teen's feelings about friends

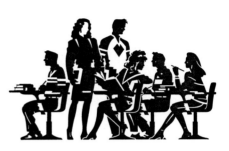

- Does your teen seem to be preoccupied with or worried about the condition of his friendships?

  Yes / No / I don't know

- Does your teen seem to have healthy friendships with the opposite sex?

  Yes / No / I don't know

- Does your teen seem generally satisfied with the quality of his friends?

  Yes / No / I don't know

- Has your teen made remarks concerning his friendships that cause you concern? Yes / No / I don't know

### Your teen's feelings about self

- Does your teen talk negatively about himself regularly?

  Yes / No / I don't know

- Does your teen seem to compare herself frequently with others?

  Yes / No / I don't know

- Does your teen seem dissatisfied or discontent with himself?

  Yes / No / I don't know

- Does your teen seem proud or arrogant concerning herself?
  Yes / No / I don't know

- Does your teen seem overly critical or impatient with others?
  Yes / No / I don't know

- Is your teen often overly critical of himself? Yes / No / I don't know

- Does your teen show signs of being a perfectionist?
  Yes / No / I don't know

## 3 Talk with Your Teen

"Nothing is as easy as talking, nothing is as difficult as communicating."[47]

It may seem that there's a lot of talking going on in your home. Listen for a moment and see if you can notice how much communication is actually taking place. For you to be able to communicate with your teen successfully, there must be a dialogue in which both parties are genuinely involved in sharing their feelings. If you or your teen don't know how to express your true feelings, then you will not experience true communication. In education, students exhibit different learning styles. Similarly, every person has a different communication and listening style. You may have a daughter that just loves to share her thoughts, then you may have a son who would rather work on his bike in silence than talk about anything "deep." Teens are notorious for giving "one-liners" in response to their parent's questions. Parents naturally use questions to try to get a conversation started. Instead of opening up with a full answer, many teens simply give responses like the following:

- "I don't know"
- "I don't care"
- "It doesn't matter to me"
- "Whatever"
- "Whatever you say"
- "So, how many miles did you walk to school in the snow?"
- "Times have changed"
- "You're not me"

- "You really don't know how I feel"
- "It's not what you think"
- "You just don't understand"
- "Yep," "Nope," "Kinda"

How many of these responses do you hear regularly from your teen? These and many other communication barriers put a halt to potential progress in the mutual communication of feelings. It takes great skill on the part of parents to get their teen to discuss honest, deep thoughts and emotions. You can actually help your teen learn communication skills by pressing them beyond their "communication comfort zone." Don't, however, put the entire burden of poor conversations upon your teen's shoulders. You can learn to draw your teen(s) out by learning certain communication skills. One skill is the sharing of your own experiences and mistakes. When shared at the right time and in the right place, this can be a powerful way of encouraging your teen to share his feelings with you. It's much more effective when communication does not come across like a pre-packaged sermon. Rather, to really draw your teen out, he must sense more of a feeling of equal footing; of growing and learning together. Your teen needs more of an adult atmosphere in the conversation because she is slowly but surely becoming one. It's of utmost importance that your teen feels secure, respected, and totally accepted during a conversation with you.

Here are some suggestions for more effective dialogue with your teen(s):

- Don't finish his sentences for him — even if he's taking too long to get his words out.

- Don't ask her, "How could you think that? Don't you know that I love you?!"

- Don't judge his comments before you have heard everything he has to say.

- Don't be critical of her choice of words while she is sharing (e.g., "Haven't I told you not to use that word?").

- Don't communicate disgust or impatience with him through non-verbal cues (e.g., sad facial expressions, defensive stances, arms crossed, toes tapping, or shaking your head back and forth in the form of a "no, no, no").

- Don't be critical of her grammar or the way she stated something while she is sharing.

The following are a few Conversation Starters to help your teen connect with his true feelings and learn how to express them to you. These also include some probing questions. After reading all of the following questions, choose which ones would be the most effective ways for you to use to begin a casual conversation with your teen. Remember that your purpose is to get your teen to open up — not shut down as a result of you dominating the conversation.

### *Feelings about God*

- *"How would you describe God? What person you know reminds you the most of what you think He's like?"*

- *"If you were to paint a picture describing the way you see God, which would represent Him the best:"*
  A. The peace and beauty of an ocean sunset
  B. The surprise and power of an avalanche
  C. The anger and devastation of a raging fire
  D. The love and tenderness of a mother for its young
  E. Some/all of the above. Explain.

- *"With as many details as possible, describe your first encounter with God."*

- *"Do you feel that you're going to go to heaven when you die? If so, how do you think that you know this? If not, would you like to know?"*

- *"Imagine that you are in heaven standing before the throne of God right now. As you stand there, God gives you an opportunity to ask Him any one question. What would your question be?"*

- *"Do you feel that you have personally experienced God's presence in your life? If so, how would you describe it to someone else? If not, would you like to?"*

- *"Have you ever felt disappointed with God? What caused you to feel that way? Has your feeling of disappointment been resolved since? If not, are you afraid that God would criticize you if you shared your disappointment directly with Him?"*

- *"Do you think that there is any difference between belonging to a religion and having a personal relationship with God? If so, what do you think the difference is? If not, could you explain your thoughts to me?"*

## Feelings about Parents and Family

- *"How would you describe the ideal family?"*

- *"What does the word 'family' mean to you?"*

- *"What is your favorite memory involving the family?"*

- *"If you had a friend who was having a hard time getting along with his parents, what would you say to him?"*

- *"If your brother or sister confided in you that he wanted to do something that you knew was not a good choice, what would you say?"*

- *"What do you think are five of your brother's/sister's greatest strengths?"*

- *"What do you think are five of your brother's/sister's greatest weaknesses?"*

- *"How would you describe the day-to-day atmosphere in our home?"*

- *"Do you ever feel misunderstood by members of our family? If so, can you give some examples?"*

## Feelings About Friends

- *"Do you have a best friend? Why is he/she such a good friend to you?"*

- *"If you had to move to a desert island tomorrow, and you had to choose only one other person to go with you, who would you choose? Would it be a family member or a friend? Why?"*

- *"On a scale of 1–10, how would you rate your social life right now?"* Explain. (1 = bad; 10 = good)

- *"What do you think is meant by the verse, 'There is a friend that sticks closer than a brother?'"*

- *"What is meant by the phrase, 'Friendship is a two-way street?'"*

- *"If the people in your life who know you the best were all sitting down together and talking about you right now, what positive things do you think they would they be saying? What negative things?"*

- *"What kind of a reputation do you think you have with your friends?"*

- *"Do you think your closest friends really know you? Why or why not?"*

- *"Do you ever feel misunderstood by your friends? If possible, give a few examples."*

### Feelings About Self

- *"So far in your life, how do you feel about the decisions that you have made? Is there anything that you would have done differently? If you can, give a few examples."*

- *"If you were to meet yourself on the first day of school, what do you think would be your first impression?"*

- *"If you could ask God anything about why He created you just the way He did, what would you ask Him?"*

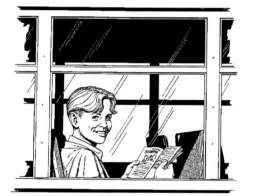

- *"If you had the power instantly to change any of your thoughts or thought patterns, would you choose to change any of them? If so, what?* (This question does not apply to changing your appearance or personality.)

- *"Do you feel that it's wrong or proud to like yourself? Why or why not?"*

- *"Do you think that it's wrong to talk positively about yourself to others? Why or why not?"*

- *"Do you know of anyone who seems to have a low or negative self-esteem? When you're around that person, how do you feel? What's your impression of that type of person?"*

- *"Do you know of anyone who seems to have a high or positive self-esteem? When you're around that person, how do you feel? What's your impression of that type of person?"*

- *"Do you think that there's a difference between being a proud and egotistical person and being a person who has a positive self-image? If so, please explain."*

- *"Into which of the following categories would you place yourself? (a) low self-esteem (b) positive self-esteem (c) proud or egotistical*

## 4 Take Action

The goal of these Action Steps is to help you tap into whatever may be causing your teen emotional turmoil. These steps are also a tool to help you talk with your teen about God, family, friends, and self.

❏ After reading this section on emotional health, list three people who you feel you would like to talk to about your teen:

- _____

- _____

- _____

❏ After listening closely to your teen, rank the following in order of their concern to you. (1 = highest concern; 2 = average concern; 3 = fair concern; 4 = little or no concern) After you rank them, start working on the area of your highest concern.

- Your teen's feelings about God _____

- Your teen's feelings about the family _____

- Your teen's feelings about friends _____

- Your teen's feelings about self _____

❑ If, after discussing your teen's feelings about God, you decide that you would like to begin a specific devotional time with your teen, use the outline below to write out the details. Afterwards, present your idea to your teen to see if he would like to do it.

- Purpose for devotional:_____

- Time it will take:_____

- When we will do it:_____

- Book to use as a guide (besides the Bible):_____

- Date we will begin: _____

- The topic with which we will begin: _____

_____

❑ Continue to pray for your teenager's choice in friends. Below, record the names of any of your teen's friends whose lives you desire to see changed by God. Next, record several positive character qualities that you would like to see in any new friend your teen makes.

- Names of your teen's friends to be touched by God:

_____

_____

_____

_____

- Positive character qualities desired in any new friend of your teen:

  _____

  _____

  _____

❏ Pay closer attention to your teen's statements about himself. Speak more positively about you teen to him. List five positive attributes of your teenager below. Compliment him about these attributes this week.

- _____
- _____
- _____
- _____
- _____

## *5* Pause to Reflect

After you finish the appropriate Action Steps, complete this evaluation to see how the chapter worked for you.

- How well did you "connect" with your teen in this section?

  Not very well        Fairly well        Very well

- After reading this section, how stable do you feel your teen's emotional health is?

  Unstable        Fairly stable        Very stable

- After reading this section and interacting with your teen, do you feel that you have a good idea of what he thinks about God?

  Yes        No        I still don't know

- After reading this section and talking with your teen, do you feel that you have a good idea of what he thinks about your family?

  Yes        No        I still don't know

- After reading this section and chatting with your teen, do you feel that you have a good idea of what your teen thinks about his friends?

  Yes          No          I still don't know

- After reading this section and talking with your teen, do you feel that you have a good idea of what she thinks about herself?

  Yes          No          I still don't know

- After reading this section, what did you learn about your teen that you didn't know before?

- After reading this section, what did you learn about yourself?

- After reading this section, what did you learn about your family?

- How successful were the Conversation Starters with your teen?

  Not very successful          Somewhat successful          Very successful

- Record any further insights, questions, or comments concerning your teen's emotional "earthquakes" here:

## Further Resources

*Preparing For Adolescence*, Dr. James Dobson, Regal Books, 1978.

*Life on the Edge: A Young Adult's Guide To A Meaningful Life*, Dr. James Dobson, Word Publishing, 1995.

*Parenting Teens with Love and Logic: Preparing Adolescents for Responsible Adulthood*, Foster Cline, M.D. & Jim Fay, Pinon Press, 1992.

*Disappointment With God*, Philip Yancey, Harper Collins, 1988.

*Hassles, Problems that Hit Home: 7 Sessions on Family and Dating*, Lyman Coleman, Serendipity House, 1994.

# The Disciplines of Time Management

*The legacy to our children will be tainted if we fail to put forth the effort necessary to develop habits of discipline... Its effects aren't immediately visible. Parents must continually remind their children, continually follow-up on them, continually pray for them. Regardless of lessons taught, they never seem to see the value of daily habits... Discipline is hard to quantify. It builds over a lifetime in small, hard-to-detect increments.*[48]

## *1* Know the Causes

As a young college student, the description about life that I came to appreciate the most came to me from one of my professors just before I graduated. She told me, "Life is like a wave which seems to be moving in to crash over you. If you don't develop self-discipline, life will control you, instead of you controlling life." When I first heard these words, I was never finding enough time to accomplish all that I wanted or needed to do. My lack of responsible time management resulted from a lack of disciplined habits. I was about to learn that an undisciplined life would produce struggle, frustration, and disappointment.

Time management is only one of the principles of disciplined living. Time is a unique resource given to each person, a resource waiting to be used wisely and productively. Time does not "stand still." Neither does it "fly by." Time is a constant, ongoing opportunity for us. Although we may feel that time is what we need the most but don't have enough of, the amount of time that we have at our disposal does not change. It's the same every day, every week, every year, and for everybody. The Bible makes is clear that we are to value the time that we have and use it wisely for the Lord:

"So teach us to number our days, that we may gain a heart of wisdom."
Psalm 90:12

"See then, walk circumspectly; not as fools but as wise, redeeming the time, because the days are evil." Ephesians 5:15,16

Responsible use of time takes good planning as well as self-discipline. You may have encountered problems with your teen in the area of assuming responsibility. An unwillingness to assume responsibility can be a selfish or lazy attitude affecting his daily life. A parent can help a teen internalize the character traits of work, commitment, and follow-through by assigning him daily responsibilities. This helps a teenager to plan his time so that responsibilities are met.

Goal-setting is an important part of time management. Setting a goal is like setting a course for the direction of one's life. If done properly, consistently, and divinely directed by God, goals can carry a person from one success to another. An important lesson that teens must learn early is that they must set goals that are consistent with the will of God for their life. You can help your teen prioritize his goals by regularly discussing how they relate to God's sense of vocation in his life. Accomplishing small goals and living a disciplined life helps teens live up to their potential and gain confidence. I've seen many teenagers with low self-esteem blossom after they began to accomplish small, realistic goals.

The following are several reasons why teenagers may not manage their time well:

- Procrastination: a learned habit that "puts everything off."

- Personality type: more care-free attitude, not strict or demanding of herself.

- Poor example: lack of quality time management at home.

- Never "made to": needs direct guidance from parents to develop disciplines; lacked having to do chores, responsibilities, and homework around the house.

- Fear of success or fear of failure: Whenever a goal is set, there's always the chance of not attaining it. When you don't, it seems like a failure. So, if you never take a risk and try, you'll never fail, right? Wrong – you fail by default. Not trying can be a failure in itself.

- Lazy: has not learned how to discipline the body to go against natural, selfish feelings.

## 2 Observe Your Teen

Whatever the reason your teen may struggle with the discipline of time management, it's never too late to set in motion positive lifestyle habits. However, what works for one teen may not work for another due to teens' varying learning and work styles. Most certainly, when teenagers can see accomplishments clearly by breaking down responsibilities into small, realistic goals, they will reap the benefits. When you observe your teen, try to notice what environment he works best in, and what seems to help motivate him.

- Does your teenager often complain about not having enough time to get everything done? Yes / No / I don't know

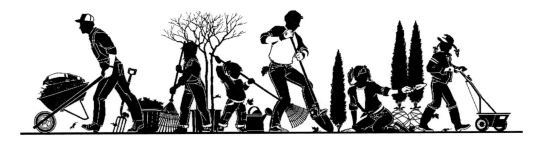

- Does your teenager need you to remind her several times about accomplishing one task? Yes / No / I don't know

- Does your teenager spend much of her time watching television or listening to music or the radio? Yes / No / I don't know

- Does your teenager openly discuss with you his goals for school and activities? Yes / No / I don't know

- Have you ever discussed goal-setting with your teenager? Yes / No / I don't know

- Does your teen regularly bring home too much homework from school? If so, do you think that it's directly related to wasted time during study hours at school? Yes / No / I don't know (If you don't know, how might you find out?)

- Is your teenager's room consistently a mess? Yes / No / I don't know

- Does your teenager consistently miss fun activities because of unfinished homework or chores? Yes / No / I don't know

- Does your teenager work well by himself? Yes / No / I don't know

- Is your teenager a procrastinator? Yes / No / I don't know

- Do you think that your teenager suffers from a "fear of failure"?
  Yes / No / I don't know

- Do you think that your teenager wastes time?
  Yes / No / I don't know

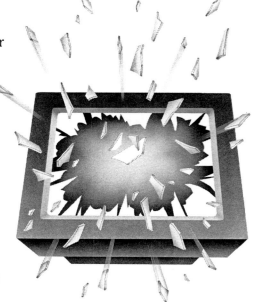

As you take a personal inventory of your teen's use of time, it's impossible to account for every hour or minute of each day. Instead, look for general patterns. As you observe her behavior at home and keep an ear tuned to what is happening at school, you may notice certain bad habits leading to regular wastes of time. Note these consistent patterns. Fortunately, a disciplined life at home will affect positively a teen's life outside the home. If your teen has developed a good habit of time management doing homework at home, it's likely that your teen will use the same discipline at school.

Although your teen has fixed commitments each day such as school, sports practice, choir, chores, and job, it's the "in-between" minutes and hours that are often wasted. The following is a sample of a fixed commitments chart. Help him fill in his fixed commitments. By keeping accurate record of how he uses free time, you and your teen can find valuable time slots that could be used more profitably.

## Fixed Commitments Chart

|        | Sun. | Mon. | Tues. | Wed. | Thurs. | Fri. | Sat. |
|--------|------|------|-------|------|--------|------|------|
| 6 am   |      |      |       |      |        |      |      |
| 7 am   |      |      |       |      |        |      |      |
| 8 am   |      |      |       |      |        |      |      |
| 9 am   |      |      |       |      |        |      |      |
| 10 am  |      |      |       |      |        |      |      |
| 11 am  |      |      |       |      |        |      |      |
| 12 pm  |      |      |       |      |        |      |      |
| 1 pm   |      |      |       |      |        |      |      |
| 2 pm   |      |      |       |      |        |      |      |
| 3 pm   |      |      |       |      |        |      |      |
| 4 pm   |      |      |       |      |        |      |      |
| 5 pm   |      |      |       |      |        |      |      |
| 6 pm   |      |      |       |      |        |      |      |
| 7 pm   |      |      |       |      |        |      |      |
| 8 pm   |      |      |       |      |        |      |      |
| 9 pm   |      |      |       |      |        |      |      |
| 10 pm  |      |      |       |      |        |      |      |

Comments:

Take the opportunity to discuss goal-setting with your teen. The following are some practical pointers that will help.

## *Principles for Positive Goal-Setting*

1. Set goals for each area of your life. Prayerfully consider your physical, mental, social, and spiritual goals.

2. Keep the goals realistic. Keep your goals attainable and do not compare them with others.

3. Word the goals in a positive way. Instead of saying, "I'll never be late for school," say, "I'll be on time for school."

4. Make a detailed plan for accomplishing each goal… and follow the plan. If your goal is to be on time for school, then your plan might be, "I will get up 30 minutes earlier than usual. I will set my clothes out the night before."

5. Make long-range and short-range goals. A long range goal may be to become a teacher or to attend college. A short-range goal might be to get a 3.0 GPA this semester.

6. Record your goals. Keep an organized book or list so you can always refer to your goals.

7. Keep your goals private. It's a good idea to share your goals with one or two significant people in your life to help keep you on track, but, generally speaking, it's better not to announce your goals to every friend you have.

8. Re-evaluate your goals regularly. Goals change just as circumstances change. Don't be afraid to adjust a goal.

9. Do it now! Your first goal should be to begin goal-setting. Get in the habit of asking yourself, "What's the best use of my time right now?"

10. Strive for excellence without becoming a perfectionist. Allow yourself some freedom. The purpose of goal-setting and time management is to relieve stress not to create it.

# 3 Talk with Your Teen

After reading all of the following questions, choose which ones would be the most effective ways for you to use to begin a casual conversation with your teen. Remember that your purpose is to get your teen to open up — not shut down as a result of you dominating the conversation.

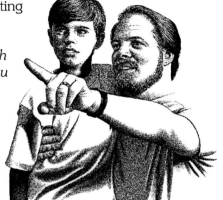

- *"Do you feel that there's never enough time in the day to accomplish all that you want to do?"*

- *"Do you ever feel like circumstances are controlling you rather than you controlling them?"*

- *"If you wanted to purchase something that you couldn't afford right now, how would you go about planning to pay for it?"*

- *"How would you describe self-discipline to your brother, sister, or friend?"*

- *"On a scale of 1–10, how would you rate your present level of self-discipline?"* (1 = poor; 10 = great)

- *"How does a teen measure self-discipline?"*

- *"Do you know anyone who manages his time very well? If so, what makes you think that he manage his time well? What kind of person is he, generally?"*

- *"Do you know anyone who manages his time very poorly? What makes you think that he manages his time poorly? What kind of person is he, generally?"*

- *"What kind of person do you want to be in five years? ten years?"*

- *"What would you like to be doing in five years? ten years?"*

- *"List one goal you have in each area of your life: physical, mental, social, and spiritual."*

- *"How are you planning to attain each goal?"*

- *"Rank the following list of fears on a scale of 1–10 in light of what you fear the most and what you fear the least."* (1 = least feared; 10 = most feared)

  _____ The fear of what others would think or say.

  _____ The fear of the unknown.

  _____ The fear of disappointing parents, siblings, friends, or others.

  _____ The fear of disappointing or hurting God.

  _____ The fear of missing God's perfect will.

  _____ The fear of others being better than me.

  _____ The fear of people saying "no" to me.

  _____ The fear of criticism.

  _____ The fear of success.

  _____ The fear of failure.

- *"Is there anything that I can do as your parent, or that we can do as a family to help you better to:*

  ❏ accomplish your goals?
  ❏ become more disciplined?
  ❏ help with time management?
  ❏ overcome fears that may hinder you from reaching your potential?"

## 4 Take Action

The goal of this time management section is to help you and your teen become aware of valuable time that may otherwise be wasted. It's to show you the importance of developing the discipline necessary to make wise use of each day. This section will also motivate your teen to develop the habit of setting short and long-range goals. It's very important that you emphasize to your teen how God wants him to begin to learn how to seek Him in establishing and accomplishing goals. The Lord does not expect teens to do everything on their own. Make clear to your teen that:

- Even if you fail at something, YOU are not a failure.

- Failure is only temporary. You will have another opportunity to succeed at something else or at another time.

- God is not in the habit of keeping a record of all your mistakes and failures.

- Failures in life can become positive learning experiences, if you let them.

- "If at first you don't succeed, try, try again!"

- After reading this section, support your teen's use of the fixed commitments chart.

❏ After observing and talking with your teen, plan a brief weekly discussion with your teen concerning his goals for that week.

❏ After reading this section, begin to counsel your teen on how to overcome some fears that you didn't know she had. Remembering the phrase: "Success breeds success."

❏ Help your teen to develop some academic goals. Encourage him to accomplish them.

❏ Back your teen in forming some physical goals. Inspire her to reach them.

❏ Stand by your teen as he comes up with some positive social goals. Contribute to his attaining of them.

❏ Assist your teen in developing some spiritual goals. Clear away all of the obstacles possible so that he will be able to arrive at them soon. (See Unit Four: Making the Spiritual Connection for more details.)

❏ Pray that the Lord will help your teen to grow in the disciplines necessary to reach the full potential that God has for him.

## 5 Pause to Reflect

After you finish the appropriate Action Steps, complete this evaluation to see how the chapter worked for you.

● How well did you "connect" with your teen in this section?

Not very well          Fairly well          Very well

● What did you learn about your teen and his time management that you did not know before?

● What did you learn about your teen's fears that you were not aware of until this time?

● What did you learn about your family as a result of this material?

● Decide to talk to the following people about your teen's time management habits away from home:

A. The following teachers at school:

_____

_____

_____

B. The parent of a good friend with whom your teen often studies or spends time

C. Extra-curricular instructors, *e.g.*, coaches, music, or drama teacher

D. Your teen's brothers or sisters who know more about his activities than you do

- Buy your teen a student calendar or organizational tool with which he can keep track of his responsibilities.

- Record any further insights, questions, or comments concerning your teen and time management here:

## Further Resources

*Raising Wise Children*, Carolyn Kohlenberger and Noel Wescombe, Multnomah Press, Portland, Oregon, 1990.

*Raising Kids Who Turn Out Right*, Tim Kimmel, Multnomah Press, Sisters, Oregon, 1993.

*Raising Kids Who Hunger For God*, Benny and Sheree Phillips, Chosen Books, 1991.

*Where There's A Will There's An A, How To Get Better Grades In High School*, Video Series, Claude Olney, Chesterbrook Educational Publishers, 1989.

*Student Success Secrets*, Eric Jensen, Barron's Educational Series, Inc., 1982.

*The Parent Connection*

# The Issue of Self-Esteem

*We draw conclusions about our appearance, physical abilities, and intelligence not only by the input we receive from others but from our own "self-talk." Our own thoughts and words have power, "For as a person thinks within himself, so is he" (Proverbs 23:7).*[49]

A teen's self-image is formed by all his past and present experiences. Many of the thoughts that teens assume others have of them are untrue. When teens assume what others think about them, they are concluding that they are a certain way whether it's true or not. When teens make such false assumptions, they actually surrender some of the power over their lives to others. They give to others the power to influence their attitudes and behavior.

A teenager's self-esteem is even more fragile than an adult's. Many teenagers feel unstable, insecure, and even unloved. In an effort to feel more loved and accepted, teens will judge themselves by how their appearance, physical abilities, and intelligence are valued by society and their peers. When teens feel that they measure up to the standards of society and their peers, they will tend to have a good self-esteem, probably superficially. When they don't feel that they measure up, then they will have a poor self-esteem — if they are not taught to have a relationship with a God who accepts them just as they are. Even though parents should encourage their teen to develop his talents and to dress clean and neat, it is even more important that they help their teen to put a higher value on the inner character of Christ. "Men judge by the outward appearance, but God judges by the heart." ( I Samuel 16:7)

# 1 Know the Causes

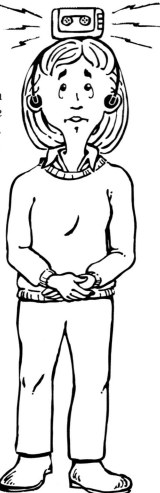

Several factors influence a teen's self-image. The most powerful influence are words. Teasing is as common as peanut butter and jelly sandwiches. Sometimes the jokes can be humorous and fun, but, most of the time, the words are hurtful and are instantly recorded in a teen's memory bank. Whoever coined the phrase, "Sticks and stones may break my bones, but names will never hurt me," did not know the emotional sensitivity of a young person.

> "But no one can tame the tongue; it is a restless evil and full of deadly poison. With it we bless our Lord and Father; and with it we curse men, who have been made in the likeness of God…" (James 3:8–9)

Unfortunately, teens remember negative input more than positive input. After awhile, their minds play back messages that they heard from their friends, and they are on the road to a poor self-image. Negative input does not only come from spoken words, it can also come from gestures, facial expressions, or silent messages from society that communicate the message, "You'll never measure up." Whatever the source, negative input can devastate an individual. What makes it worse for teenagers is that they have a deep need for acceptance. Teenagers easily turn the input that they receive from others into their own "self-talk." Self-talk is the tape that runs in a person's head. It repeats to them all of the positive or negative words that they have ever heard, seen, read, or imagined. When teens allow themselves to believe the negative "untruths" that they hear, it affects their relationships, attitudes, and behavior. Teens cannot control what others will say or do to them, but they can learn how to respond to what they hear from a Christian perspective. There's great power in the Word of God to help erase a teen's negative self-talk.

# 2 Observe Your Teen

Use the following exercise to see if your teen suffers from negative self-talk.

- How often does your teen criticize himself?

  Not often          Somewhat often          Very often

- Rank the following three categories according to the most prevalent content in your teen's self-talk. ( 1 = most often heard; 2 = occasionally heard; 3 = least often heard)

  ___ physical appearance ("I'm ugly." "I'm skinny." "I'm fat.")

  ___ physical abilities ("I'm not good at anything." — whether it be athletics, music, drama, computer, academics, art)

  ___ intelligence ( "I'm so stupid." "I'm not good in any of my classes.")

- Do you believe that your teen knows how to transform the negative input he receives into positive input?

  Not at all          Sometimes          Most of the time

- How often have you heard other family members negatively tease your teen-ager?

  Not often          Somewhat often          Very often

- Does your teen demonstrate a general lack of self-confidence in the way that he carries himself, i.e., how he stands, walks, or talks?

  Yes / No / I don't know

- How often does your family speak positively to and about your teenager?

  Not often          Somewhat often          Very often

- How often does your family use the Word of God to help build each other's self-image?

  Not often          Somewhat often          Very often

- In general, what kind of self-esteem do you believe that your teen has?

  A negative self-image        An average self-image        A very positive self-image

- Do you believe that your teen needs to hear more positive messages about himself? Yes / No / I don't know

The other day, I was driving my oldest son, Steven, home from kindergarten. "How was school today?" I asked. He responded quietly, "The boy who sits across from me told me that he thought that the picture that I had colored was ugly." I replied, "What do you think of your picture, Steven?" As he looked at his pink gingerbread man, he said, "I kinda like him." "I like your picture, too, Steven," I stated, trying to reinforce my son's positive self-talk about his own picture. "What did your teacher say about your picture?" I inquired, looking for another source of positive feedback. "She said it was great. See the sticker she put on it!?" Glad at hearing Steven's positive note, I tried to bring out the moral of the whole incident, "Does it really matter what that boy thought of your gingerbread man if the most important people — you, your teacher, and your Mom — like it so much?"

Steven is only five years old, and he has a long road ahead of him. The long road of caring what others think doesn't change too much even well into the teen years. Very similar to young children, teenagers, too, are consumed by what others think of them. They are often afraid of being who they really are out of a fear of being criticized or rejected. Driven by their desire for acceptance, teens usually spend far too much time concentrating on their physical appearance and far too little time focusing on their inward character qualities. The fact is that most teens have a deep respect for those who have a strong self-image.

> "Most teenagers respect a guy or girl who has the courage to be his own person, even when being teased." [50]

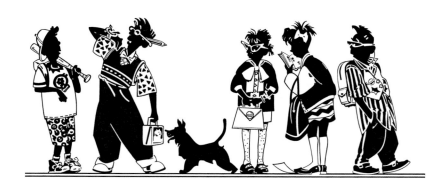

# *3* **Talk with Your Teen**

After reading all of the following questions, choose which ones would be the most effective ways for you to use to begin a casual conversation with your teen. Remember that your purpose is to get your teen to open up — not shut down as a result of you dominating the conversation.

- *"How do you feel about your appearance?"*

- *"Are there certain aspects of your appearance that are impossible for you to change? If so, in what way would you try to help yourself to accept them?"*

- *"Are there aspects of your appearance that you know you have the power to change? If so, what could you do about them?"*

- *"What physical skills or abilities do you know that you have? How do you feel about them?"*

- *"What talent or skill would you like to have someday? How do you think that you would go about learning that skill?"*

- *"How do you feel about your intelligence level or desire to learn?"*

- *"Who has ever hurt your feelings by what they said to you? What was it that they say to you? How do you feel about those comments today?"*

- *"Who has ever made you feel really good by what they said to you? What was it that they said? How do you feel about those comments today?"*

- *"What do you think is meant by the verse, 'God created man in His own image. In the image of God He created him. Male and female He created them?'"* (Genesis 1:27)

- *"Do you think that Genesis 1:27 could affect your life in a positive way? If so, how?"*

- *"Do you know a person who has poor self-esteem?"*

- *"What would you say to a friend who always seemed to talk negatively about himself?"*

# 4 Take Action

The goal of this section on self-esteem was to help you gain better understanding of your teen's feelings about himself. It may also open the door for deeper communication about your teen's deep feelings about how he thinks about himself in his mind, his "self-talk."

❏ After reading this section, have you concluded that your entire family needs to increase its encouragement of your teen's self-image? If so, rank the following options in the order that you feel your teen needs the most amount of self-esteem work. (1 = the area of greatest self-esteem need; 4 = the area of least self-esteem need)

\_\_\_\_\_ appearance
\_\_\_\_\_ physical abilities
\_\_\_\_\_ intelligence
\_\_\_\_\_ character qualities

❏ If your teen has a problem in the area of his physical abilities, plan for you or your spouse to work closely with him to improve his desired skill level, e.g., basketball, volleyball, music, drama, auto, speech, art, computer.

❏ If your teen needs help with his physical appearance, teach him self-acceptance skills simultaneously with trying to bring desired personal improvement through the following: acne medicine, weight control ideas, a few newer outfits, weight-lifting for your son, a little make-up for your daughter, a fun make-over.

❏ If your teen needs help with academics, here are a few ideas: plan for your teen to get help after school from the appropriate teacher; buy some learning aids or educational computer programs; hire a tutor (maybe an older student who would like a little extra spending money); or, you or your spouse help him yourself according to your own academic skills.

❏ Write out a few pertinent scriptures and give them to your teen to help overcome his negative self-talk. **Nave's Topical Bible** can help you here.

❏ Consciously try to control your own negative self-talk so as to set a good example in your home. Be open with your entire family about how you are working to increase your positive self-talk. Your teen will respect you for this.

❑ Encourage your teen to develop the inward character qualities that make anyone naturally attractive, e.g., humility, kindness, friendliness, joy, helpfulness, and a listening ear.

❑ If you feel that your teen's self-esteem is dangerously low — resulting in deep depression, contact a professional Christian counselor immediately.

## *5* **Pause to Reflect**

After you finish the appropriate Action Steps, complete this evaluation to see how the chapter worked for you.

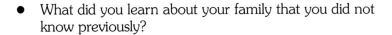

● After doing the Action Steps that you felt were right for your situation, how would you describe your teen's self-esteem now?

Low Fair        Good           Excellent

● How well did you "connect" with your teen in this section?

Not very well          Fairly well        Very well

● What did you learn about your teen that you did not know before?

● What did you learn about your family that you did not know previously?

● What did you learn about yourself that you did not know before?

- How well did this section's Conversation Starters work with your teen?

  Worked poorly          Worked fairly well          Worked great

- Record any further insights, questions, or comments about your teen's self-esteem here:

## Further Resources

*By Design, In God's Image, Self-Esteem from a Judeo-Christian World View*, Dr. Larry G. Day, Mt. Tabor Press, 1992.

*Raising Positive Kids in a Negative World*, Zig Ziglar, Thomas Nelson, 1985.

*His Image....My Image*, Josh McDowell, Here's Life Publishers, 1984.

*Building Your Self-Esteem*, Josh McDowell, Thomas Nelson.

*The Five Cries of Youth*, Merton Strommen, Harper and Row, 1974.

*The Five Cries of Parents*, Merton Strommen and Irene Strommen, Harper and Row, 1985.

*The Tongue, A Creative Force*, Charles Capps, Harrison House, 1976. Further Resources

*None of These Diseases*, S.I. McMillen (Fleming H. Revell, division of Baker Book House, 1984).

*Talking with Your Kids about the Birds and the Bees*, Scott Talley, (Ventura: Regal Books, a division of Gospel Light Publications, 1990).

*Preparing for Adolescence,* Dr. James Dobson. (Ventura: Regal Books, a division of Gospel Light, 1989).

# SOCIAL HEALTH

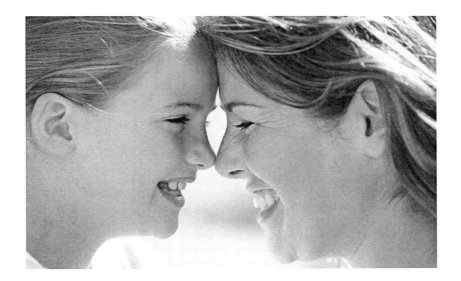

*You are the world's light – it's impossible to hide a town built on the top of a hill. Men do not light a lamp and put it under a bucket. They put it on a lamp-stand and it gives light for everybody in the house. Let your light shine like that in the sight of men. Let them see the good things you do and praise your Father in Heaven.*

*Matthew 5:14–16, Phillips translation*

# Teens Learning Responsibility

*Do you want freedom without responsibility? That combination will not work.*
*If a person is not yet ready to accept all the responsibilities of living, then he is*
*not ready to handle unrestricted freedom either.*[51]

Teenagers' desires for freedom and independence expand the older they become.
They have strong feelings about receiving ever-increasing amounts of unrestricted
and unsupervised space. One thirteen-year-old put it this way:

> "It all comes down to independence, and this lack of independence probably
> causes most of the problems between teens and their parents. Independence to
> me is being able to do what I want to do, when, and how I want to do it. One
> thing I know is when I do get this independence, my world will expand."

Yes, a teenager's world will expand when he is given more independence. With every gradual "expansion," however, wrong choices will be made and lessons will have
to be repeated. At present, do you think that your teen has the necessary attitudes,
character, and convictions to make his step into independence a responsible one?
Along with their natural desires for independence, parents need to impart to their
teens a serious awareness concerning increasing responsibility. With every increase
in personal freedom, there is an increase in personal responsibility. How your teen
balances out freedom and responsibility will ultimately determine his maturity level
and success in life.

What follows is a list of some of the basic responsibilities that God has given to
Christians. You can use this list as a discussion guide with your teen.

### Responsibilities as a Christian:

- Love and seek God (Deuteronomy 6:5; 2 Corinthians 5:14).

- Love and serve others (1 Peter 1:22).

- Extend God's kingdom by sharing the gospel of Christ (Matthew 28:19; Mark 16:15).

- Obey God's commandments (Deuteronomy 10:12,13; 13:4; 30:8,16).

- Be a good example in word and deed (1 Timothy 4:12).

### Responsibilities as a Person:

- Physical: take proper care of your body ( I Corinthians 3: 16–17;  I Timothy 5:23).

- Mental: increase your professional training and education, according to your calling and resources (Matthew 25: 24–28). Though not indicative of your teen's heavenly reward, such training may be a means of fulfilling his divine destiny as well as influencing society for Christ.

- Social: love others sincerely, with heartfelt emotion (Romans 13:8–10). Since God is in the "people business," so is your teen.

- Family: love, respect, serve, and obey in the home (Ephesians 6:1–4).

### Responsibilities as a Citizen:

- Showing responsibility for the environment (Leviticus 25:1–7).

- Being a responsible and educated consumer and business person (Proverbs 22:26; 11:1; 20:14; 31: 14,18,24).

- Preparing to be a responsible citizen in the country in which one lives (Romans 13:1–7; I Timothy 2:1–3).

Parents are to train their teen(s) to be responsible in every area of life. The principle of being faithful in little before you are given more is a good motto for teens (Matthew 25:21). Teens must prove that they can carry the responsibilities that come with entering into the world of a young adult, by taking care of smaller duties first.

"Freedom is not really valued for its true worth unless it is earned."[52]

# 1  Know the Causes

Responsibility is a heavy word. If your teen, however, has been taking on bite-size pieces of responsibility throughout his life, the teen years will not seem to be unbearable. The biggest freedom that understandably brings concern to parents is the handing over of the car keys to their teen. If your teen has not learned respect for others, dependability, and cautiousness before he receives privileges to the family car, it will be a time of worry, nagging, sharp words, power struggles, and frustration for the whole family. When teens get legal permission to drive alone, they instantly feel a new surge of independence. When teenagers obtain their driver's license, they commonly think, "This is it. I've arrived. I can now do anything that I want to." Such a moment genuinely tests all of the values and convictions that you have worked so hard to instill in your teen during preadolescence. All that you have taught him suddenly goes on the line. From that point on, generally speaking, your teen's real convictions will primarily be tested out from under your protective eye.

As far as a teen's development chart is concerned, getting to drive a car is like a teen experiencing a huge physical growth spurt. Driving is a gigantic jump from one trust level to another; an enormous move from one level of responsibility to the next. Consequently, the best way that a parent can prepare himself and his teen for such a juncture is to let out the line slowly every year so that it will not be a sudden, unknown experience. Impart and repeat the character qualities necessary for such privileges to be given. Parents who decide that their teen is not yet ready for such a responsibility should communicate to their teen exactly what he needs to develop in order to earn the privilege that he desires so strongly. Also, it should be made very clear that the same privileges that have been given can just as easily be revoked or suspended if abused. To ensure your teen of being able to drive or assume other major preroga-tives that he desires, continually challenge him to maintain the high standards which you have taught him (see I Timothy 4:6).

## 2 Observe Your Teen

Answers to the following questions will help you to understand your teen better in this area.

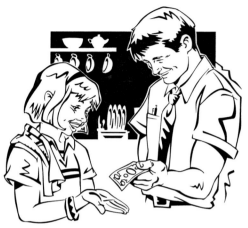

- Over the years, has your teen increas-ingly earned more freedom and inde-pendence? Yes / No / I don't know

- Are you satisfied with the amount of responsibility that your teen has shown in your home up to now? If not, in what areas do you think that he should improve? Yes / No / I don't know

  Needs improvement in: _____ _

  _____

- Does your teen consistently obey the rules of your household?
  Yes / No / I don't know

- How does the thought of your teen getting his driver's license make you feel?
  Extremely worried    Naturally concerned but confident    No particular feeling

No parent can know for sure how his teen will handle greater freedom and re-sponsibility. It's important, however, that a certain element of trust be shown every step of the way. When your teen acts responsibly and uses his freedom wisely, you should increase the level of trust that you have in him. If your teen makes a mistake (which I am sure he will do sometime) don't panic or allow yourself to feel like a failure. Give grace where grace is due, and always use mistakes as teachable moments to impart lifelong lessons.

If you feel that your teen is just not ready for the responsibilities that many of his peers are gaining, then you make the call. Maybe he should not be allowed to get his license until demonstrating more character over a longer period of time in a certain area. As a parent, even when you think that you can take a deep sigh of relief and relax for a while, you'll realize that your teen will continue to need your input and your boundaries. If you need help in talking with your teen about your expectations concerning freedom and responsibility, use the following Conversation Starters.

## 3 Talk with Your Teen

After reading all of the following questions, choose which ones would be the most effective ways for you to use to begin a casual conversation with your teen. Remember that your purpose is to get your teen to open up — not shut down as a result of you dominating the conversation.

- *"What do you think it means to be responsible?"*

- *"Do you have a friend who you feel is a very responsible person? What makes you think that he is responsible? What kind of person is he? How much freedom is he allowed by his parents?"*

- *"Do you have a friend who you feel is very irresponsible? What makes you think that she is an irresponsible person? What kind of person is she? How much freedom is she allowed by her parents?"*

- *"Which of these two friends would you rather hang around? Why?"*

- *"Do you feel that you're a responsible teenager? In what ways do you feel this?"*

- *"How can a teenager earn more freedom? How can you personally earn more freedom?"*

- *"What kinds of expectations do you feel from us, your parents? Do you feel that our expectations are too high for you?"*

- *"What kinds of expectations does God place on all of His children? Do you feel that God's expectations for us are too high? How do you think that God expects us to be able to do all the things that He asks us to do?"*

- *"If you were eligible to get your driver's license today, would you feel that you had earned this freedom and privilege? Why or why not?"*

- *"If you were going to take your driver's license test today, how would you describe some of the feelings that would probably be going on inside of you? What kinds of feelings do you think would be going on inside of me? Let me tell you…."*

- *"Besides a driver's license, what other freedoms do teenagers earn as they mature?"*

- *"What do you think is meant by the quote, 'God has a special plan for everyone. No one can stop it, but many can miss it?'"*

## 4 Take Action

The goal of this section on responsibilities is to help you evaluate whether your teen is ready for more freedom and independence. As teens mature, their parents should increasingly involve them in the decision-making processes that they use to determine their teen's boundaries and limitations. Such involvement — as long as it's sincere and not token — will enable teens to feel less and less like little children. They will also feel that their parents trust them. It should be easy to get teenagers to talk when they know that what they say might mean that their parents would give them more of the freedom and independence that they want.

❏ After reading this section, do you feel that you should give your teen more independence than he has had up until now? If so, how much more independence do you think that you should give him?

A lot more     A little more          Wait and see

❏ After reading this section, have you come to the conclusion that your teen is not ready for more independence? If so, which of the following best describes your reason?

- lacks a general sense of responsibility
- has abused privileges too much
- lacks basic good character

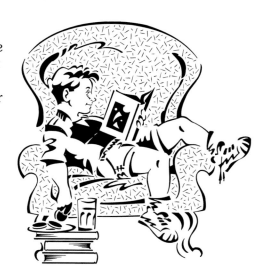

- has a poor, apathetic attitude
- other: _____

❏ Do you feel that you need to limit/cut back on your teen's present freedoms in your home because your teen is taking advantage of them? If so, in what area do you want to start cutting back and why?




❏ Do you think that you and your spouse need to have a long discussion with your teen about his need to take responsibility more seriously? If so, what would you plan on saying?




❏ Do you think that you and your spouse need to have a discussion with your teen in which you make your expectations of his behavior and attitudes inside as well as outside of your home more clear to him?

❏ Are you or your spouse confused in any way as to what to do to establish healthy responsibilities for your teen?

❏ If you feel the need, plan on seeking the counsel of one or more of the following people:
- one of your trusted adult friends: _____
- your teen's youth leader: _____
- the pastor of your church: _____
- a counselor from your teen's school: _____
- a qualified Christian counselor: _____

❏ Pray regularly that God will give you wisdom and direction in how to handle your teen and her desire for more independence.

## *5* **Pause to Reflect**

After you have finished the Action Steps, use the following questions to evaluate the effectiveness of this section in your teen's life.

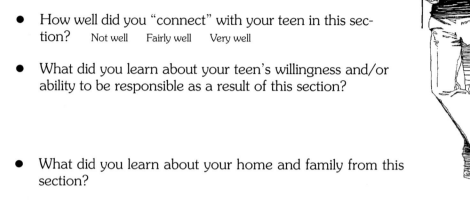

- How well did you "connect" with your teen in this section?    Not well    Fairly well    Very well

- What did you learn about your teen's willingness and/or ability to be responsible as a result of this section?

- What did you learn about your home and family from this section?

- What did you learn about yourself and your parenting from this section?

- Rank the following categories of responsibilities according to your teen's present strengths and weaknesses. Explain each of your rankings so that you will have a clearer picture of what you will do about each and in which area to start. (1 = weakest responsibility area; 10 = strongest responsibility area)

    ____ Responsibilities as a Christian. Explanation:

    ____ Responsibilities as a person. Explanation:

_____ Responsibilities as a family member. Explanation:

_____ Responsibilities as a citizen. Explanation:

_____ Responsibilities as a student. Explanation:

_____ Responsibilities as a team player. Explanation:

_____ Responsibilities as a student body member. Explanation:

_____ Responsibilities as a friend. Explanation:

_____ Responsibilities as a church/youth group member. Explanation:

_____ Responsibilities as a _____. Explanation:

- Record any further insights, questions, or comments concerning your teen and responsibility below:

## Further Resources

*Preparing For Adolescence*, Dr. James Dobson, Regal Books, 1978.

*Raising Wise Children*, Carolyn Kohlenberger and Noel Wescombe, Multnomah Press, Portland, Oregon, 1990.

*Raising Kids Who Turn Out Right*, Tim Kimmel, Multnomah Press, Sisters, Oregon, 1993.

*Raising Kids Who Hunger For God*, Benny and Sheree Phillips, Chosen Books, 1991.

CHAPTER SEVENTEEN

# Making Wise Choices

*We need to take a look at our children's world and the choices they must make. The problems of their generation are light-years removed from our own childhood dilemmas. During those years we got by quite well with a few simple*

*directions (cross with the light, don't take candy from strangers, don't smoke, don't swear, and be kind to animals). But the complex problems kids face today cannot be solved by simple rules and simple thinking. Times have changed. Lifestyles have changed. And the future has changed for all of us.*[53]

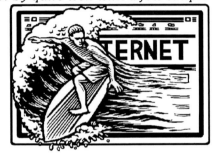

## *1* **Know the Causes**

"It's just not fair! Why do guys have it so easy, and girls have it so tough?", bemoaned one of the students of my sophomore girl's health class. Instantly, all eyes fell on me. How was I, the health teacher, going to respond to a complaint like that? I waited for a moment to collect my thoughts. I then turned to the chalkboard and wrote the name "EVE." The entire class of girls laughed, and we continued our discussion. When Eve ate the forbidden fruit in the garden, all the pain and suffering of the human condition began (Genesis 3).

> "If Eve's future rested in the hands of a judge in an American court today, she would certainly get off with a light sentence. After all, she was naive. The poor woman had fallen into a bad crowd. She had no record of previous offenses. But, God didn't save Eve from the consequences of her actions. Instead, He handed down the maximum penalty because He knew Eve had been prepared to make a wise decision. She had been given the knowledge to do what was right. The choice was hers. And she chose to eat the fruit." [54]

The human brain is a highly complex organ. It's God's crowning glory to the human creature. Its functions are endless, and its importance is immeasurable. Among its countless functions, your brain has the capacity to: store information, draw conclusions from that information, send messages of feeling and sensation to your body, cause body movements, make difficult decisions, and aid you in discerning between right and wrong. To equip us more fully to discern between right and wrong, God has placed in all of us a conscience. Our conscience is the home where the Holy Spirit resides and guides us.

God created all of us with free will. All human beings have the power to make their own choices. Everyday we must live with the consequences of our decisions. Our choices range from pressing or not pressing the snooze button on our alarm clock in the morning to whether we eat pepperoni/sausage pizza or a salad for dinner. Decisions are an inescapable part of life. Sometimes our choices are decisions by commission, other times they are decisions by omission or even default. The phrase, "Not to decide is to decide" bears some deep thought. One of the problems with teens is that they have a tendency to feel indestructible and unmoved by the consequences of their decisions for various reasons. One reason is that teens don't always experience the negative consequences of a poor decision immediately. E.g., they may get away with cheating on an exam at school; they may break the speed limit in their car, not get a ticket, and no one get hurt; they may lie and no one expose it; they may smoke some pot in private, feel euphoric, and not get addicted to anything harder; they may sleep with their boy/girl friend and not catch a STD or not result in a pregnancy. Because of these facts, some of the additional points to communicate to inquiring teenagers about choices and consequences are:

- Even if a consequence cannot be seen immediately, it does not mean that it doesn't exist or that it won't be experienced eventually.

- Even if a consequence cannot be seen outwardly, it doesn't mean that it cannot be felt internally.

- Even if a consequence can't be seen by people outside of the situation, it doesn't mean that it isn't being felt by those inside of the situation.

- There are many different kinds of consequences — not just one, e.g., spiritual, personal, vocational, marital, emotional, physical, familial, financial, legal, ecclesiastical, social, political.

- Consequences can be experienced at different times. Some consequences for bad behaviors (including rewards for good behaviors) won't be experienced until the final Judgment Day (I Timothy 5:24; Revelation 14:13).

- If a teen decides to continue a poor decision based on the fact that, so far, he/she has not received any negative consequence from it, it's very possible that they will develop life and soul threatening habits over time.

> We live in an "instant" society... But this "right now" mentality can be dangerous... Right choices, on the other hand, often require waiting for better long-term results. [55]

How can we help our teens make right choices? We can help them to make correct decisions by setting clear boundaries for them from the very beginning: "Don't touch that lamp," "Don't go into the street." Parents set these types of boundaries for their children for their own safety and good. Teens need to understand that God does not place boundaries in their lives so that He can watch them fail or rob them from having fun. God sets boundaries to protect teens and to give them a longer, healthier, and more fulfilling life. God is a loving Father who is trying to protect His teenage children from harm and danger. How can you better prepare your teen for the difficult choices ahead? You can prepare your teen to make wise choices in the days that lie ahead by:

- helping your teenager overcome peer pressure,

- teaching him always to look ahead at the possible future consequences of a decision,

- encouraging your teen to value a clear conscience above all else,

- being consistent, when necessary, with the consequences that the Lord has asked you to bring to bear upon your teen's life.

# 2  Observe Your Teen

Does your teen presently demonstrate the ability to make wise choices? What is his decision-making record? Read the following observations to see how mature your teen's decisions are.

- Has your teen consistently shown the maturity necessary to make wise choices? Yes / No / I don't know

- Does your teen have a sensitive conscience? Yes / No / I don't know

- Has your teen used wisdom in the friends that she has chosen?
  Never    Sometimes    Often

- Have you talked with your teen concerning how to make wise choices?
  Never    Sometimes    Often

- Have you talked with your teen concerning the consequences of wrong choices?    Never    Sometimes    Often

- Is your teen a positive influence on his peers?    Never    Sometimes    Often

- Does your teen seem to have a strong devotional life? Yes / No / I don't know

- Does your teen respect both of his parents? Yes / No / I don't know

- Does your teen stand by her convictions?
  Never    Sometimes    Often    I don't know

- Does your teen consistently avoid compromising situations?
  Never    Sometimes    Often    I don't know

- How often is your teen a leader rather than a follower?
  Never    Sometimes    Often    I don't know

- How often does your teen speak up for what is right?
  Never    Sometimes    Often    I don't know

- What do you think that your teen would do if he was found in a compromising situation where the pressure to conform was extremely great?

Leave　　Hang around out of curiosity　　Join right in with the group　　Try to redirect the group

## 3 Talk with Your Teen

Unfortunately, a teen's good intentions will not prevent him from making mistakes. Sometimes the consequences are minor, and sometimes they are life-altering. Often, teens don't know how to discern what may very well be "a trap arranged by a serpent-in-waiting."[56] Discernment is the ability clearly to recognize the inner nature or true intention of a certain person or situation. When teenagers possess discernment, they are able — mentally and spiritually — to distinguish good from evil. Such an inner ability to understand spiritual and moral reality results in sound judgments. So, how can you help your teen to develop this valuable spiritual commodity? You can begin by talking with your teen and listening very closely to his reasoning process. A good way of hearing your teen's thinking process is to use the case study approach. In the case study approach, you ask your teen, "In such-and-such a situation (here describe either a true or hypothetical situation that bears directly upon the topic you want to talk to them about), what would you do and why?" Then listen very carefully.

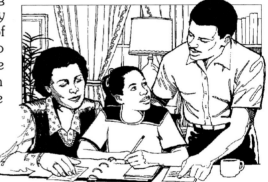

After reading all of the following questions, choose which ones would be the most effective ways for you to use to begin a casual conversation with your teen. Remember that your purpose is to get your teen to open up — not shut down as a result of you dominating the conversation.

- *"Have you ever been asked to do something that you knew would make you compromise your convictions? If yes, what decision did you make?"*

- *"Have you ever been in a group where certain teens were trying to get you and others to watch something or go somewhere when you knew you shouldn't? What did you do?"*

- *"Would you describe any of your peers as a follower? What makes you think that he's a follower? What is this person like to be around?"*

- *"Would you describe any of your peers as a leader? What makes you think that he's a leader? What is this person like to be around?"*

- *"Have you ever done something with the thought in your mind that you would do it 'just once'? If so, what happened? How did doing whatever it was 'just once' make you feel? Did you come away from that situation with any conclusions? If so, what were they?"*

- *"Have you ever confronted someone who did or said something that you didn't think was right? What did you tell the person? How did you approach them? How did that person respond? How did it make you feel?"*

- *"How would you describe the kind of an influence that most of your friends have upon your spiritual life?"*

- *"How would you describe the kind of influence that you have upon the spiritual lives of your friends?"*

## 4 Take Action

The goal of this section on discernment is to help you observe your teen's present capacity to make wise choices. The following Action Steps will help you to train your teen in this essential life skill by assisting him to put wisdom before curiosity.

❏ After reading this section on making wise choices, write notes and letters to your teen encouraging him to make wise choices.

❏ Write some hypothetical situations on some 3 x 5 cards. Have your teen pick a card and then explain to you what he would do in that situation. If any dialogue or role-playing could be involved and the subject is appropriate, you can make the situation into a skit and involve the entire family.

❏ Have your spouse share his/her point of view with your teen concerning making wise decisions.

❏ Have a discussion with your teen about what it means to "avoid the appearance of evil" (1 Thessalonians 5:12). If you want to make the discussion go deeper, ask the question, "Did Jesus obey the principle of avoiding the appearance of evil when He ate and drank with some of the local prostitutes?"

❏ When you're talking with your teen(s) about sexuality, you might want to ask them, "If sex in marriage is good and God created it, why does the Bible not contain any 'how-to' book on the subject? The only 'guide' we have is the Song of Songs."

❏ Pray regularly that God will give your teen wisdom in her thinking processes and decisions. Also pray that He will give you wisdom to guide your teen in the making of right choices.

❏ Ask your teen if he believes that there are any areas in your own life in which you are not making very wise decisions.

## 5 Pause to Reflect

After doing whatever Action Steps you feel are appropriate for your teen, you can evaluate this section's overall success with the following questions:

● After reading this section and observing your teen, do you believe that he has the ability to make wise choices?

● How well did you "connect" with your teen in this section?

   Not very well      Somewhat      Very well

● What did you learn about your teen that you didn't know before?

- What did you learn about your parenting style from this material?

- What did you learn about your spouse's parenting style from this chapter?

- How well did the Conversation Starters work with your teen?

  Not very well     Somewhat     Very well

- Record any further insights, questions, or comments concerning your teen and wise choices here:

## Further Resources

*Right From Wrong: What You Need To Know To Help Youth Make Right Choices*, Josh McDowell and Bob Hostetler, Word Publishing, 1994.

*Preparing For Adolescence*, Dr. James Dobson, Regal Books, 1978.

*Raising Wise Children*, Carolyn Kohlenberger and Noel Wescombe, Multnomah Press, Portland, Oregon, 1990.

*Raising Kids Who Turn Out Right*, Tim Kimmel. Multnomah Press, Sisters, Oregon, 1993.

*Raising Kids Who Hunger For God*, Benny and Sheree Phillips, Chosen Books, 1991.

*Choices, Dare To Be Different, 7 Sessions on Lifestyle*, Lyman Coleman, Serendipity House, 1994.

# More Than Just Saying "No" to Sex

*...In order to help teens effectively avoid premarital sexual involvement, parents must begin early teaching and demonstrating wholesome, godly sexual values and attitudes. When Christian values, attitudes, and accurate information are provided in an atmosphere of openness and love, children will be much less likely to succumb to sexual temptations. Our energy should be concentrated on providing positive, ongoing sex education for our children.*[57]

In all the books, tapes, and articles that I've researched on the subject of teens and sexuality, I was unable to find anything that said, "Christian teenagers never engage in sexual activities." I cannot write a section on sex and promise that if your teen believes in God and what the Bible says about premarital sex, that he/she will absolutely not engage in sexual activities. During my years teaching at a Christian school there was one thing I noticed — teens will be teens — no matter if they're Christian teens or not. Since all teenagers are experiencing intense hormonal changes in their bodies, all will have thoughts and temptations that come with adolescence. The scary fact is that Christian young people have a great tendency to hide what they are truly feeling. For different reasons, they are often afraid to share with their parents for fear of disappointing them. They're afraid of talking to a teacher for fear they will be "exposed" — publicly or otherwise. The factor that makes teenagers more open to talking about their sexual struggles is an open, honest, and accepting atmosphere in the home. No school, church, youth group, or Bible camp can do for your teen what you must do at home.

"A relationship. Acceptance. Security. Self-esteem. Knowing they are loved and can love others. Every teenager must have these needs met, and we as parents play a vital role in meeting them for our children. Giving our children a relationship, acceptance, security, a healthy self-esteem, and letting them know that they are loved and can love others is far more important than giving them money, educational opportunities, a family reputation, or presents. If they don't get love at home, they will seek it outside the home." [58]

If parents "lay down the law" with their teens concerning sex but have not developed a strongly positive relationship with them as the foundation, the result is usually devastating. Josh McDowell puts it so well: Rules without relationship lead to rebellion! All of your rules against sex without an open and healthy relationship with your teen will probably lead either to his active resistance or passive indifference to all that you have said.

# 1 Know the Causes

The following are questions and comments I have heard from teenagers concerning sex. I follow each with some ideas as to how parents might respond.

- **"I know all I need to know about sex."**

It's common that teenagers believe they know all they need to know about sex. I taught a class of sophomore girls about menstruation, ovulation, conception, and birth. The minute that the girls walked out into the hallway, I knew that I was in trouble. The girls immediately began to chatter, "Today in class, we learned about SEX!" The next day in class I raised the question, "How would you define the term 'sex'?" The class proceeded to give me at least ten different responses. Before class was over, I had them record my definition of this loaded word: "Sex is the activity that arouses the desire for more sexual activity with the intended end being intercourse." After the girls had written my definition into their class notes, I posed to them this question, "Yesterday, when we talked about menstruation, ovulation, conception, and birth, were we talking about 'sex'?" They all responded with an unanimous, "No."

If your teen claims that he knows all that he needs to know about sex, I would proceed to ask your teen how he defines sex. When you teach about abstaining from sex, are you saying abstain from intercourse, or abstain from anything that arouses the desire for more sexual activity? Does your teen understand what your value of moral purity really means? Does your teen have any moral purity values in his life?

- **"All I want to know is, how far is too far?"**

One day I taught a session to my health class on abstinence. In the middle of my lesson, a female student raised her hand and bluntly asked, "All I want to know is how far is 'too far'?" "You will hear different answers to this question," I responded. Inside of my heart I was hoping that this girl was not trying to find someone who would let her get by with sexually doing just as much as she wanted. Unfortunately, that's the attitude of a lot of people — including teenagers. People will continue asking various authority figures in their lives the same question until they find someone who gives them the answer that they want to hear. It's usually an answer that's as close to the border of sin/pleasure as possible. Too many teens "go too far" without going "all the way," i.e., they justify their engagement in sexual activity on the basis that they are not having intercourse. If you, or your teen, hold the view that it makes no difference how far teens go sexually just as long as they don't "go all the way," I'd like to challenge you...

> "...[teenagers] pride themselves on having refrained from intercourse. Sexual experience is gained, but virginity is preserved. This kind of activity is so widespread that a new term has been coined by psychologists and counselors to describe the teens in this category....[The new term is] "technical virgins"... Biblically speaking, they are observing the letter of the law but not its spirit. Since the Bible forbids only sexual intercourse anything but intercourse is considered fair game (in the teen's mind)." [59]

Though giving us a shocking but necessary insight about the term "technical virgins," let's look a little more closely at the end of Talley's quote, "Since the Bible forbids only sexual intercourse anything but intercourse is considered fair game (in the teen's mind)." Honestly, I find this statement somewhat misleading because it gives the impression that the Bible does not forbid any other type of sexual focus or activity before marriage except intercourse. This simply isn't true.

First, we have Jesus bringing the idea of purity from just the outward act into the realm of the heart and the mind. One of the cornerstones of moral purity from Scripture is Christ's own standard. Jesus defined moral purity on a much deeper level than just the act alone. To Jesus, if a man inwardly lusted for a woman, he had already committed adultery with her in his heart.

Jesus said, "You have heard that it was said, 'You shall not commit adultery;' but I say to you, that every one who looks on a woman to lust for her has committed adultery with her already in his heart. And if your right eye makes you stumble [causes you to sin], tear it out and throw it from you; for it is better that one of the parts of your body perish than for your whole body to be thrown into hell. And if your right hand makes you stumble [causes you to sin] cut if off and throw it from you; for it is better for you that one of the parts of your body perish, than for your whole body to go into hell." (Matthew 5:27–30)

Second, the Bible forbids all sexual licentiousness. Licentiousness is sexual license or excess (Galatians 5:19; Romans 13:13; 2 Corinthians 12:21). "Evil concupiscence" is also forbidden (Colossians 3:5). In its root, concupiscence means to "breathe heavy," thus to stimulate or be stimulated sexually. So, sexual stimulation outside of marriage is forbidden by the Bible.

Third, the word that is used for "fornication" in the NT not only condemns sexual intercourse outside or before marriage. It also condemns "every kind of sexual transgression."

Fourth, communicate to your teen that being a Christian means more than observing the letter of the law. The Bible teaches us to live by its spirit and underlying principles (1 Thessalonians 4:3–7; Galatians 5:16–19). Certainly, for two teenagers to get each other sexually stimulated before marriage (when they cannot legitimately consummate such excitement with intercourse) is not only wrong but unfair and defrauding. It stands clearly against the spirit of the Bible and of Jesus Christ Himself.

What should a parent do who realizes that genuine moral purity is more than just stopping before one goes "all the way?" The most important thing that you can do is to instill in your teen Christ's view of moral purity before he's ensnared in a moment of passion. If you do, you will save his entire life from much pain, disappointment, guilt, and struggle. Again, we're not trying to quench a teen's growing natural attraction to the opposite sex. We're simply encouraging you to instill in your teen the biblical value that sexually stimulating activity with the opposite sex before marriage is forbidden fruit. One of the metaphorical meanings of "fire" in the Bible is sexual activity outside of marriage (Proverbs 6:27). Robertson wrote, "The man who plays with fire will get burnt." We have to remember that the teen who plays with sexual fire before marriage will also get burnt!

## • "I have the self-control to stop at anytime."

"I understand that the purpose of sexual stimulation is to culminate in intercourse, but I have self-control. I know that I can stop at anytime." This is a common feeling that many people have. Unfortunately, overconfidence reveals naiveté and sets up for a fall.

When a teenager tells me that he has "total control," I know that he doesn't know what he's talking about. All human beings do reach sexual "points of no return" because God created sexual stimulation to operate that way in the context of marriage. Such braggadocio statements reveal immaturity, inexperience, and extreme naiveté. A teen's extreme vulnerability to immorality at such a young age is clearly highlighted in Paul the apostle's warning: "While other sins must be overcome by spiritual crucifixion of the flesh (Galatians 5:24), the sin of immorality (porneia) is one from which the Christian must flee in order to keep pure (I Corinthians 6:18)."[60]

It's because of a fundamental fact of nature that Paul gives this warning about avoiding sexually compromising situations. It's clear from nature that the normal, natural, and God-ordained direction of all sexual stimulation is intercourse. Therefore, if the sexual stimulation cannot lead to a legitimate end in marital intercourse, then what teenager has the right to start the process of lovemaking? It's off limits. They're trespassing. These statements are built upon the scriptural belief that true moral purity means more than just abstaining from intercourse. We must tell it to our teens straight: sexual arousal leads to intercourse and this is only allowed in marriage.

Along with our honesty about the dangers of sexual stimulation before marriage, however, I also believe that we are obliged to share the positive side of abstinence; give them something to look forward to when they get married, the joy of sex in marriage. So, to me, the question is not about pushing the edge, seeing how far I can go without reaching the point of no return, or, seeing how much I can get away with. The real question is why do 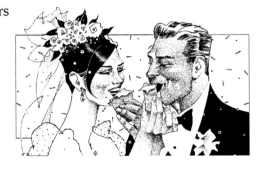 Christian teenagers feel that they have the right to sexually stimulate each other before marriage when it's clear that all sexual stimulation is to be reserved for the joys of reaching a legitimate and beautiful marital consummation?

- **"But I don't feel guilty for doing it."**

Furthermore, besides attempting to educate your teen's conscience with scripture, I recommend that you teach your teen not to violate his conscience. Even though not violating one's conscience is somewhat of a subjective call, keeping self-consciously consistent with ones inner self is a sure way to stay mentally and emotionally healthy. Obviously, one teen's conscience will be more sensitive than another's; possibly, some girl's conscience's will be more sensitive than some guy's. But this is a healthy and scriptural principle to teach your teen because if your teen allows himself to violate his conscience, even a little, he'll be more likely to violate it again, a little more. It becomes easier for a teen to allow himself to "go a little farther" each time he indulges in sexual pleasure.

You can also share with your teen the fact that Christianity is all about doing whatever is best for the highest good of the other person. So, if your teen's body is feeling sexually aroused, he should know that the person he is with is also experiencing similar — if not stronger — feelings. Selfishly pushing someone else beyond the boundary of his personal conscience is part of what it means to defraud someone; to arouse sexual desires in another which cannot be righteously satisfied; and righteously means only in marriage. Just as your teen's conscience is not the final standard, neither is one's friend's conscience. In any couple, there can always be one who is looser and another who is more scrupulous.

To experience God's greatest blessings, however, all consciences must ultimately submit to the standard of God's word; a word which forbids teen couples, or any other couples for that matter, to stimulate one another sexually outside of the marriage covenant. As to the sacredness of this covenant context, the writer to the Hebrews wrote, "Marriage is to be honored by all, and marriages are to be kept undefiled, because fornicators and adulterers will come under God's judgment." (13:4, Jerusalem Bible)

> "Selfish use of others for personal gratification violates the basic message of Christianity." [61]

- **"Why does God give teens such strong sex drive when He doesn't allow them to fulfill it?"**

In biblical times, many couples married in their teens. In today's society, however, young people usually wait until they're out of college and/or secure a good job before they get married. This delay prolongs the years of dating, courtship, singleness, as well as sexual temptation. In one sense, a sexually alive teen could ask why God allows this. Is there any advantage sexually in postponing marriage until, very typically, one's latter twenties? Yes, it's learning self-control. Teens need to gain some perspective on sex and marriage. Communicate to your teen the fact that just becaus a person gets married doesn't n all sexual temptations cease — especially if a teen has been promiscuous. Promiscuity has a tendency to breed promiscuity — even after marriage.

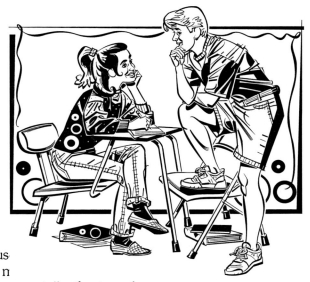

Once a teen's hormones have tasted the sugar pop, as it were, they instinctively want more. Postponing marriage and sex trains young people in the self-discipline that they will need, but don't see as yet, after they get married. Another aspect of self-control that the delay brings is in the male. Typically, married men want sex more frequently than their wives. In delaying his sexual fulfillment until marriage, it will only help a man to be able to have more self-control when he is married and may not be able to enjoy the intimacy as often as he would like. God wants teens to learn self-control now so that after they are married, their self-discipline will have been so ingrained that they will have the character in both mind and body to keep a marriage together and happy. A lasting relationship is built on more that just sex. Love, respect, and commitment are even more important. Generally speaking, sex (physical intimacy) is the easiest part of marriage. What really takes work (and what will make the sex even better) is the ability to give of oneself so as to experience emotional, intellectual, and spiritual intimacy.

- **"I've already lost my virginity, so what difference does it make now?"**

Virginity is only part of the picture. Saving yourself for the right person is still the goal. Why add sin to sin or guilt to guilt? In order to be emotionally healthy, a teenager must feel like the atmosphere in his home is one of grace, mercy, and forgiveness. After all, grace, mercy, and forgiveness is what Christianity is all about through Jesus Christ. Such is the love of the Father toward all of us. Yes, God feels grieved when teens compromise their convictions, but his mercy and forgiveness toward them is unending. Teens who have lost their virginity can experience God's mercy, regain their moral strength, and pursue moral purity more strongly than they ever did before when they come to Jesus for forgiveness.

When teens make mistakes and only receive judgment and condemnation from their parents, they will tend to view God as also unable or unwilling to forgive them. This is a tragedy. An inability to repent of sin, have guilt removed, and walk on in faith will cause teens to grow up with a core of shame inside. They will constantly have a deep, nagging insecurity in the core of their being that constantly tells them that God doesn't love them; they aren't good enough; and that they'll never measure up. This shame will only lead them to more failures and a downward cycle away from God. Remind your teen of David's mistakes but how God still used him mightily because he sincerely repented (Psalms 51).

- **"But, what if I'm in love?"**

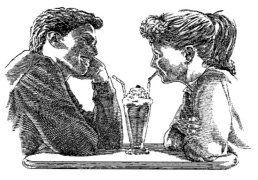

Teenagers have a misunderstanding about true love. Television, movies, romance novels, and music lead them to believe that love is an emotion and is demonstrated through the giving of sexual permission. They mistake a superficial, emotional infatuation for a lifetime committed relationship. Josh McDowell explains it this way:

> "The biblical picture of love is one of giving without expecting anything in return, of accepting without conditions, and of security in a relationship without performance. A lack of understanding about real love usually results in confusion about sex and love. Granted, they should go together in the right context, but they are not synonymous. They are two separate concepts. Sex is an act performed by two people committed to loving each other for life, while love, in varying degrees, can be felt by anyone. Love is not an act; love is a commitment." [62]

- **"What was your honeymoon like?"**

It's a fact. Teenagers are curious about sex. After my husband and I returned from our honeymoon, some overly-curious girls in my health class asked me, "Well, what happened? Tell us what your honeymoon was like!" The moment that I heard their questions, I knew that the girls didn't want me to bring out our travel brochures and tell them all about all of the sights and sounds that we had seen on our trip. They wanted to know about sex. "What was it like to have sex? What does it feel like? Is it as great as people say it is?" In answering their sexual queries, I had to choose my words very carefully. On the one hand, our honeymoon was absolutely none of their business, but on the other hand, I didn't want to lose a "teachable moment" and send them away with a smug and self-righteous feeling. Such teen curiosity about sex is normal, it is very important that parents make sure that their teens get their information from the proper sources.

> "Parents…. should assume the responsibility of educating their kids about sex and regulating what they are exposed to. This does not mean children should be sheltered, but it does mean there needs to be open, frank discussion about the sexual messages and images adolescents receive so that their curiosity will be satisfied by their parents. One of the ways this curiosity can be satisfied is to let young people know their parents enjoy sex… let them see you enjoying hugs and kisses with your mate and to verbalize that you enjoy being close…. Our goal as parents is not to keep sex among teenagers unknown, just unexplored."[63]

- **"It'll never happen to me."**

Does your teen view himself as indestructible? When my thirteen-year-old nephew, John, first turned on his Sega Saturn system, it sounded quite fascinating. Running furiously past monsters, over deep canyons, and through jungle trees, the game that he was playing, Sonic the Hedgehog, sounded like a lot of fun. Every now and again, however — sometimes all too often — his "guy," Sonic, would "die," and then he would have to start the game all over again from the beginning. It was quite frustrating to John when Sonic "died." One day, however, I was told that something had changed. Sonic the Hedgehog never "died." He just kept going and going resplendently through all of the obstacles he encountered. Even through the game's toughest sections, Sonic never, ever "died." This definitely piqued my curiosity. I wanted to know why, when I first heard about Sonic, he died fairly frequently, but, later, he never "died." Why? What I was told was very enlightening. John had simply made Sonic "invincible." He had made Sonic unable to "die" by purchasing a game accessory called, Game Genie. With Game Genie, a teen can do all sorts of neat maneuvers with his "guys" that he couldn't do without it.

When John told me how making Sonic "indestructible" made him feel, this is what he said, "Making my 'guy' invincible is so cool. I can sit there and keep racking up more and more points without any obstacles stopping me. That's what you do when you use the 'invincibility' option: you must rack up points. When I use the 'invincibility' code, I feel that I can do whatever I want to do!"

Like their simple entering of the "invincibility" code in Game Genie, many teenagers feel that nothing bad will ever happen to them. Because young men believe that they'll never get injured, they partake in risky activities (including speeding in their parent's cars). Because young women believe that they'll never get pregnant, they become promiscuous and end up contracting an STD or even AIDS. Teens with this fairy-tale attitude don't think very long about the potential physical consequences to their sexual activities. They may even be so naive that they believe they will never find themselves in a sexually compromising situation. They overconfidently assert, "Don't worry about me, Mom and Dad, I would never do that."

Teens need to know that even though they have this feeling like nothing bad can happen to them, it's mostly because of their young age, lack of true life experience, and feeling of hope and health. Somehow teens need to come to believe that bad things can and do happen to young people just like themselves. And, unfortunately, for reasons which we do not fully understand, tragically bad things do happen to sincere Christian teenagers. Teens need to understand that many things, obviously, are totally beyond their own control (being hit by a drunk driver, being approached by a teacher). But one area that's definitely within their control is not putting themselves in potentially sexually compromising situations. True, being morally pure begins with teens keeping their thoughts, literature, movies, jokes, and conversations pure. What also helps is a sense of reality about one's own weaknesses. Just when teens think they are impervious to sexual sin, they find themselves weak. Teens are not expected to handle sexual pressure on their own. Every parent knows that from his/her own experience from being a teen. Teens need a strong support system at home as well as regular avenues through which they can receive God's grace.

- **"I believe in abstinence, so why won't my parents let me single-date?"**

Whenever I heard a teenager tell me that he was determined to make abstinence his choice, I was thrilled. Nevertheless, I always pressed him/her to be more specific by presenting them with a scenario. "Let's imagine that your parents let you date the great Christian guy who you have had your eyes on all year. After your date is over, he drives you to the top of a hill overlooking the city lights. The view takes your breath away. After a bit of light conversation, he puts his arm around you. You feel so happy that he likes you and is showing you so much attention. You trust him and don't even think about the possibility that he might try to go further. Then, all of a sudden, he leans over and kisses you. You're quite surprised, but you go along with it because it makes you feel beautiful. Besides, you think, he's a strong Christian guy with good character. The kisses and the feelings between you intensify, and soon he begins to touch your breasts. You tell yourself that it's OK — after all, he's only touching the outside of my blouse. At the same time, he's thinking that you won't mind if he goes a little bit further because you haven't raised any objections so far. After some time passes and both of you are sexually turned on, this "great Christian guy" now wants to go all the way. He says that he loves you. He says not to worry because he brought a condom in his pocket. So, this was the innocent date for which you begged your parents? Why did it turn so sour? What are you going to do now? ….What should you have done?"

Teens need to be challenged from their very early years to avoid compromising situations like this. Part of what will help to motivate a sincere teen not to put himself into similar compromising situations is understanding their sexuality from God's view point. God did not give teens their sexual desire as an evil craving, or a source of unending frustration. Their sexual desire is good, healthy, and normal. The Lord wants them to be acutely aware, however, that their sexual desire is a very powerful engine that was not meant to be shut down once it got legitimately going. After being legitimately fired up on their wedding night, their sexual motor will bring them a lifetime of joy and satisfaction in marriage.

Sexual arousal was meant to be progressive. A little arousal is supposed to lead to more arousal. God made it that way. How else would babies be brought into the world? God did not make each teen's sexual motor to be turned on and off like a light switch. The key to sexual fulfillment for every teen, however, is not allowing their sexual motor to be turned on while they're single. It was meant to be turned on only in marriage and then it would take them to a good destination. For their own good, we don't want our teens to get their sexual motors fired up and feel guilty about doing what is totally normal and natural to do in the right context. Out of its proper context, sex becomes guilt-ridden and destructive. In its God-ordained context, sex is innocent and beautiful.

Another way to try to ensure that your teen avoids potentially sexually compromising situations is to involve him in a discussion about limits and boundaries. If you allow your teen to single date, here are a few ideas that you can use to begin a good discussion on this subject. A general principle is stated first, followed by some questions that you can ask your teen.

- Never let your daughter single date someone that both you and your family don't know very well.

  **Questions to ask your teen:** How well do you want to know someone before you single date him/her? What are some good ways to get to know someone before you single date him/her? What are some inadequate ways of getting to know someone?

- On single dates, have your teen always avoid being totally alone with his/her date.

  **Questions to ask your teen:** Where are you going on your date? Are those the only places you're going? What are some places that some people go to be alone or to kiss? Would you want to take your date there "just to talk?" Who else will be going with you? What do their parents say about their dating activities?

- On single dates, avoid sitting and talking alone in the car.

  **Questions to ask your teen:** Where will you be parking your car for this date's activity? Where can you talk in semi-privacy without talking alone in your car?

- Develop a mutually agreeable boundary for physical contact.

    **Questions to ask your teen:** Have you developed a standard for physical contact on dates? If so, what is it? Do you feel that it will be hard or easy to keep to that standard? With this person, what do you feel about: holding hands? a kiss on the cheek? kissing on the lips? kissing on the lips for a long time? French kissing?

## 2 Observe Your Teen

Now that you have read a few of the thoughts that Christian teenagers have about sex, answer the following questions concerning your teen(s) to help you find out if you understand what he/she may be thinking and feeling.

- Have you and your spouse had any significant conversations with your teen about sexual arousal, petting, and intercourse?   Yes   No   Plan to soon

- Have you and your spouse had any significant conversations with your teen about sexual boundaries, setting clear standards for what is appropriate physical contact on dates?   Yes   No   Plan to soon

- If your teen hasn't already genuinely accepted your sexual boundaries and dating standards, how open do you think that he will be to them when you discuss the subject?   Very open   Probably defensive   Somewhat open   I don't know

- If you don't think that your teen is very open to your sexual boundaries and dating standards, why do you think that is?
    - ❏ a strong will?
    - ❏ poor communication on your part?
    - ❏ unwillingness to talk on teen's part?
    - ❏ sexual sin in teen's life?
    - ❏ lack of good sex education on our part?

- Have you heard your teen verbally express his commitment to abstinence from premarital intercourse as his choice?

    Yes   No   I don't know   Plan to ask soon

- Has your teen verbalized a personal commitment to abstain from all sexually arousing physical contact before marriage?

    Yes   No   I don't know   Plan to ask soon

- Have you talked with your teen about what the Bible means when it forbids us to sexually defraud one another?

  Yes  No  I don't know    Plan to ask soon

- From the categories previously covered, check any option below that you feel fits your teen. What follows each category parenthetically is what you might want to work on with your teen if you checked that box.

  ❏ "What is your definition of sex?" (may need to review the difference between sexual "plumbing" [physiology] and natural sexual response [emotion, touching, and arousal] )

  ❏ "How far is 'too far'"? (probably has not set sexual boundaries or formed specific dating standards; may be privately violating standards already set)

  ❏ "I can stop any time I want." (may not understand the phenomenon of weakening one's own or someone else's conscience; may be experientially naive and in need of learning about the reality of "points of no return")

  ❏ "Why did God make me with such a strong sexual desire, if He won't allow me to fulfill it? 'It's just not fair' attitude." (probably needs to work seeing the joy of sex in marriage as something to look forward to; work on presently disciplining his/her sexual desires; realize that his/her strong sexual feelings are universal; learn the power of sublimation)

  ❏ "If I believe in abstinence, why won't my parents let me single date?" (may need to review how to screen for a trustworthy date; may need to read some articles about the reality of date rape; may be helped by reviewing facts of natural sexual response [emotion, touching, and arousal]; review how to avoid potentially sexually compromising situations)

  ❏ "I've already lost my virginity, what's the use?" (needs to know how to repent and receive mercy and forgiveness personally from a loving God; may need to see God as more loving and kind — less harsh/judgmental; may need parents to repent of judgmentalism toward him/her; may need to understand that many falls are much worse than only one; may need hope for the future — that he/she hasn't ruined his/her future for a happy marriage)

  ❏ "But I'm in love, why not?" (needs to know the difference between love and sex, commitment and infatuation; needs to know how 'used' girls feel after they go all the way and then get dumped; needs to understand the typical male response to a girl who sleeps with them: inward loss of respect, more easily break up, use "I love you" only to get sex, stay together only for sex)

❏ "What was your honeymoon like?" (may need to ask parents sex questions to satisfy curiosity; may need to know difference between "plumbing" [physiology] and sexual response)

❏ "It won't happen to me. The 'I'm indestructible' attitude." (look at his/her past failures to see human weaknesses; needs to read or hear about those who got pregnant or contracted a STD or AIDS that had the same attitude; may need further instruction in reality of natural sexual response [emotion, touching, and arousal]; may need more discussion of the frequency of sexually compromising situations )

● What do you believe the atmosphere in your home is mainly like?

Rules and the law    Relationship and love    Attack/defend    Openness/honest sharing

● Do you honestly believe that your teen feels that if he told you that he were no longer a virgin, or that your daughter informed you that she was pregnant, that you and your spouse would be loving and forgiving?

Yes / No / I don't know

● Do you believe that your teen would come to either you or your spouse if he engaged in premarital sex? Yes / No / I don't know

● As far as you know, has your teen:

❏ ever been kissed? Yes / No / I don't know

❏ ever engaged in petting? Yes / No / I don't know

❏ ever had intercourse? Yes / No / I don't know

❏ ever looked at pornography or seen sexual activity in a movie?

Yes / No / I don't know

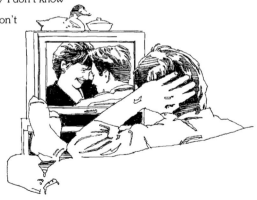

● If you asked your teen about all of the points in the previous question, do you feel that he would answer you honestly? Yes / No / I don't know

# *3* Talk with Your Teen

If Christian parents want to hold to a higher moral standard than what they see in society, then open and honest dialogue with their teen must be a priority in the home. Evaluate the plan you have to help your teen to live a sexually pure life. Having a plan is really best because it's so easy to allow time to pass, and then before you know it, an issue catches you by surprise. It will help if you tried to imagine what you would say or do in any scenario. Prepare yourself to see your teen frustrated with your high standards. Remain strong but understanding. Keep reinforcing how the benefits of moral purity outweigh the physical pleasures of the moment.

You may find that some of the Conversation Starters in this section are too heavy for you and your teen right now. If you do, only ask the ones with which you are most comfortable and then move on from there. Don't be afraid to go into this area of sexuality. Some parents hesitate and then it's too late. Keep shining the light of God's holiness and purity because you're in a huge spiritual war for the soul of your teen. God will give you wisdom, and your teen will probably be glad you finally brought up the subject. After reading all of the following questions, choose which ones would be the most effective ways for you to use to begin a casual conversation with your teen. Remember that your purpose is to get your teen to open up — not shut down as a result of you dominating the conversation.

- *"How would you define the term sex?"*

- *"How far is 'too far' in your mind when it comes to sexual activity?"*

- *"Do you know any of your peers who have 'gone all the way?'"*

- *"How would it make you feel if you heard that your best friend had had intercourse? What would you say to him/her?"*

- *"Have you set any sexual boundaries or dating standards for yourself concerning sexual activity?"*

- *"Society keeps giving us the message that abstaining from intercourse until marriage is unnecessary and unrealistic. What is your opinion?"*

- *"If you found yourself in a compromising situation, and you ended up having intercourse, would you feel that you could tell either one or both of your parents? Why, or why not?"*

- *"If you found yourself in a compromising situation and you ended up violating your convictions about sexual activity by going farther than you thought was right (without having intercourse) would you feel you could tell either one or both of your parents? Would you want to tell them? Would you think it would help you to talk it over? What do you think that they would say or do?"*

- *"What would you say to the person who gave you the following one-liners?"*

  - ❏ "If you really love me, you'll have sex with me."
  - ❏ "If you don't have sex with me, I won't go out with you anymore."
  - ❏ "Everybody's having sex. What's wrong with you?"
  - ❏ "No one will ever find out that we slept together."
  - ❏ "People were right; you really are a prude."
  - ❏ "Since we really love each other and plan to marry someday, it's OK to make love now."
  - ❏ "We've already gone this far; why don't we just go all the way?"
  - ❏ "Your parents have too much control over you."
  - ❏ "You're old enough to make your own decisions."

- *"If your best friend asked you why it's important to you to wait to have sex until marriage, what would you say to him?"*

- *"If your best friend asked you how you handle your strong sex drive and your need for physical closeness, what would you tell him?"*

- *"If your best friend told you that he/she had just had intercourse and didn't know what to do, what would you recommend for him/her to do? Would you recommend that he/she talk with someone? If so, who?"*

- *"What do you think is the greatest challenge to teenagers?"*

## A Word About Masturbation

This subject is not covered in the student textbook. Please use this section at your own discretion.

The subject of masturbation is very controversial. I address the issue in **The Parent Connection** because I have had many students ask me if I felt that it was morally wrong. This subject is pertinent to girls as well as to boys. A question about masturbation was raised first in my girls' sophomore health class. So, if you have a daughter, don't skip over this subject. Dr. James Dobson, who has dealt with teenagers for many years, says this about masturbation:

> "Masturbation is the act of rubbing your own sex organs in order to get that same tingly feeling that you would have if you were participating in intercourse. Most boys do this sometime during adolescence, and so do many girls. Unfortunately, I cannot speak directly for God on this subject, since His Holy Word, the Bible, is silent at this point. I will tell you what I believe, although I certainly don't want to contradict what your parents or your pastor believes. It is my opinion that masturbation is not much of an issue with God. It's a normal part of adolescence, which involves no one else. It does not cause disease, it does not produce babies, and Jesus did not mention it in the Bible. I'm not telling you to masturbate, and I hope you won't feel the need for it. But if you do, it is my opinion that you should not struggle with guilt over it."[64]

Though very wise, Dr. Dobson is not the final word on every subject. You and your teen are probably going to have some heart-to-heart talks on this one. This may just be the subject for you to open up to your teen and admit to him how confused or uncertain you are about it. Your teen will always respect and appreciate you for your honesty. From my observations with Christian teenagers, masturbation is a question for which teens really want a clear answer. Their intense desire to have an answer on this rather controversial subject may be one of their first opportunities in life to seek the will of God for themselves and become "fully persuaded in their own mind" (see Romans 14:5b). It's amazing sometimes, but open and humble teens can hear from God, too! Personal conscience becomes a crucial issue in a matter such as this.

Here are a few of the comments that I have made over the years to teenagers and their parents about masturbation that seemed to have been of some help to them in their various situations:

- One person told me that she never had a problem with masturbation until she heard about it. Out of curiosity she engaged in self-stimulation, and it has been a problem ever since. She wishes she had never found out about it in the first place.

- Sometimes the more we talk about something and the bigger deal we make about it, the more it remains on our minds and the more difficult it is to stop it.

- Anytime anything becomes the constant focus of your thoughts, it's unhealthy. No teenager or adult should feel consumed with thoughts of masturbation. This act would be unhealthy if it became a daily compulsion/obsession. Paul the apostle said, "All things are lawful for me, but not all things are profitable. All things are lawful for me, but I will not be mastered by anything. Food is for the stomach, and the stomach is for food; but God will do away with both of them. Yet the body is not for immorality, but for the Lord; and the Lord is for the body." (I Corinthians 6:12–13)

- It's interesting to recall God's original intention when He created sex. He created sex to be shared between two covenanted people. Let's assume, for example, that it was God's will for both Mark and Judy — both single — to marry someone sometime. If Mark's or Judy's masturbation actively hindered either one of them from pursuing marriage, then it would be unhealthy because it was hindering God's will. Similarly, if Tom and Karen were married and masturbation by either of them actively hindered the sexual/emotional intimacy that was the will of God for their marriage, then it would also be undesirable. In light of the fact that masturbation is a solo act, some would consider it selfish and, therefore, wrong.

- An important question to ask when we talk about anyone masturbating is: Why does he/she masturbate? Is it simply to relieve the sexual tension built up hormonally in the body, and, probably doing it without fantasizing? (In my opinion, this was the thought that was behind Dr. Dobson's permission statement above.) Or, is it because he/she is fantasizing about having sex with another person? Is he/she masturbating with the use of pornography or X-rated videos? (In the latter two instances, I personally feel that the masturbation has gone too far.) Does he/she not know how to release frustration any other way? Is it because no one has ever told him that regular physical exercise can help to sublimate strong sexual tensions? These are all important questions that need to be addressed by *everyone's* conscience before the Lord.

# 4 Take Action

The goal of this section is to equip you with the tools necessary to discuss factual and relevant teen issues concerning sex. Don't feel overwhelmed. The books that are listed under the Further Resources section are excellent resources for further reading.

❑ Plan to have another talk with your teen concerning sex.

❑ Choose books and do further reading on this subject.

❑ Find out from your teen's high school teacher what is being taught on this subject and plan to sit in on the class.

❑ Do a Bible Study with your teen on moral purity (ask your teen's health teacher for the one in the *Total Health Teacher's Edition* if it is not going to be used).

❑ Have your spouse share his/her point of view concerning sex and abstinence.

❑ Pray regularly that your teen has a strong conviction concerning abstinence.

❑ Ask your teen if he anticipates marriage positively or negatively, Why?

# *5* **Pause to Reflect**

After doing whatever Action Steps you feel are appropriate for your teen, evaluate this section's overall success to you by answering the following questions:

- After reading this section, do you believe your teen has a strong personal conviction concerning abstinence? Yes / No / I don't know

- How well did you "connect" with your teen in this section?
  Not very well     Somewhat     Very well

- What did you learn about your teen that you did not know before doing this section?

- What did you learn about your parenting in this area?

- What did you learn about your spouse's parenting in this area?

- How well did the Conversation Starters work with your teen?
  Not very well     Somewhat     Very well

- Record any further insights, questions, or comments concerning your teen and his standards of sexual behavior here:

# Further Resources

*Right From Wrong: What You Need To Know To Help Youth Make Right Choices*, Josh McDowell and Bob Hostetler, Word Publishing, 1994.

*Talking With Your Kids About the Birds and the Bees*, Scott Talley, Regal Books, 1990.

*Sex, Love ,and Romance*, Hugh F. Pyle, Abeka Books, 1989.

*How To Help Your Child Say "NO" To Sexual Pressure*, Josh McDowell, Word Publishing, 1987.

*Raising Them Chaste*, Richard C. Durfield & Ranee Durfield, Bethany House, 1991

*Too Close Too Soon*, Jim Talley & Bobbie Reed, Thomas Nelson, 1990.

*Straight Talk for Guys*, Bill Sanders, Fleming Revell, 1995.

*Guys and a Whole Lot More, Advice For Teen Girls on Almost Everything,* Susie Shellenberger, Fleming Revell, 1994.

*Against the Tide, How to Raise Sexually Pure Kids in an "Anything Goes" World*, Tim & Beverly LaHaye, Multnomah Press, 1993.

*The Teenage Q & A Book*, Josh McDowell and Bill Jones, Word, Inc.

*The Love Killer*, Josh McDowell and Bob Hostetler, Word, Inc.

*It Can Happen To You* (a book on date rape), Josh McDowell, Word, Inc.

*Don't Check Your Brains At the Door*, Josh McDowell and Bob Hestetler, Word, Inc.

*Pure Excitement*, Joe White, Focus on the Family Publishing, 1996.

# CHAPTER NINETEEN

# "Mom and Dad, I'm Pregnant."

*Perhaps every parent struggles with the subconscious fear of their children engaging in premarital sex. Oh, there are those who court the idea that, "My kids are above average. I've taught them better and they're not really involved." They resist the thought that it may happen to them. But down deep most parents are concerned that their children will become sexually active, and, I believe, suffer with this same subconscious fear. It's tragic, but the fact is that your own son or daughter, your grandchild, your friend's child, or some of the kids at your church are sexually active on a consistent basis. And, if one of them becomes pregnant, what will be your attitude? What will you say? What action will you take?*[65]

## 1 Know the Causes

When an unmarried daughter finds herself pregnant, it not only affects the parents, it also affects the siblings. I observed this in my family of origin. In June, 1994, my oldest sister, Kathy, asked her two younger sisters, Ann and myself, to go with her when she told Mom and Dad that she was pregnant. When Mom and Dad saw all three of us walk into the kitchen together to talk with them, they knew something was serious. After we all came into the kitchen, Kathy confessed, "You know, Mom and Dad, I love you very much. I wouldn't do anything intentionally to hurt you. But, I'm pregnant, and I'm very sorry...." As Kathy shared her situation with our parents, I could see the deep disappointment on their faces. After a few minutes of "I can't believe it!" and, "Why didn't you use some protection?!" a feeling of hope filled the room when my Dad said, "You know, Kathy, we'll get through it."

I was very proud of my Dad for not banging his fist in rage or telling Kathy she knew better. At that point, what good would any of those words have done? It was just "water under the bridge." Over the next few months, everyone in the family was trying to sort out his/her thoughts and feelings. As it turned out, my parents allowed Kathy to live with them after she had the baby, who she named, Shaina. To be honest, during the three years that Kathy and Shaina lived with Mom and Dad, there were some very fun moments, but there were also some very tense ones. From observing what happened in my own family, I think that it's absolutely imperative that a family work together when one member faces a dilemma. Great strength and support can come from within the family, and we all need it at times.

## 2  Observe Your Teen

We have already discussed some of the reasons why teens may engage in pre-marital sex. I would hope and pray that if your daughter became pregnant that she would feel that you and your spouse would be the first people she would tell. Having a teenage daughter tell her parents first is very important for the whole family because it establishes an important context of love and understanding necessary to process all of the challenging feelings that will ensue. The following are some of the different emotions I saw my sister, Kathy, experience as she faced her unplanned pregnancy. Most, if not all young women in Kathy's position, have to learn to process the same feelings. And, they can do that best with the support of a loving God and family.

- **Anger:** anger at the man involved, anger at God, anger at herself for letting it happen.

- **Denial:** "The pregnancy test must be wrong." "I can't believe this happened to me."

- **Grief:** feeling disappointed over losing control over her own life and destiny.

- **Loss:** feeling deprived of her own freedom, her choices, her self-image, her reputation, her relationships, her future.

- **Shame:** "What will people think of me now?" "Will there be a man who will want to marry me with a child?" If not processed properly, shame can cloud every aspect of a single mother's life, i.e., work, school, caring for her child, working in the church, counseling, helping others, attending church, dating others, and relating to God.

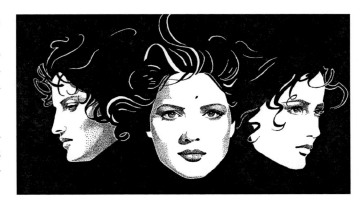

- **Depression:** feelings of hopelessness and sometimes despair.

The young, pregnant woman is not the only one who experiences these challenging emotions. Other members of the family feel them, too. Moms and Dads ask themselves, "Where did we go wrong?" Siblings feel frustrated that they can't do more to help "fix" the situation and make everyone happy again. This is a time when everyone needs the help of qualified counselors. If not a professional Christian counselor, everyone needs at least someone who will listen to how they are feeling. One Dad put it this way:

> "The next few days after learning of my daughter's pregnancy was one of the most emotional and confusing times of my life. Rarely do I shed tears, but that week I wept bitterly every day. I found myself negatively reacting to the entire situation. If it had not have been for dedicated counselors at the Crisis Pregnancy Center urging me to follow two very crucial principles, I would have probably driven my daughter to despair. These principles are:
>
> 1.   The power of forgiveness can untangle the emotional pains and clarify the thinking, and,
>
> 2.   "Committing the future to God can provide a sense of direction." [66]

## *3* Talk with Your Teen

The following letter, written by a Dad whose unwed daughter became pregnant, is the best way that I have found to comfort parents concerning an unplanned pregnancy in their family.

> "No matter which alternatives are considered, premature marriage, single parenting, or adoption – they are all painful and appear unacceptable. Confusion becomes the order of the day. Yet, when I found the power to forgive, I

gained not only a supernatural supportive love for Amy, but a clarity of heart and mind to understand the alternatives. As my emotions untangled, I sat down and wrote her a long letter. Following are excerpts from that letter." [67]

Dear Amy,

I know that during this past week you have suffered pain like never before, the burden that you bear is perhaps the heaviest you've ever carried. Yet through it all God assures us: "My grace is sufficient for you, for power is perfected in weakness" (2 Cor. 12:9).

And one thing I've come to realize is that God has not declared that life is over because of an unplanned pregnancy. God has great plans for your future. You have not been disqualified from the race. In fact, He plans to draw you closer to Him and teach you to know Him better than you have ever known Him before. Once we realize that our main purpose in life is to know God and glorify Him, life comes into proper perspective. And I believe, Amy, the more you and I know Him and see life from His perspective, the more life and all its struggles and problems begin to be resolved.

God has an answer for this situation. He has a solution. One without pain and suffering? Probably not. Yet, he has plenty of grace, that when appropriated to our lives, will be for our good and His glory. But, I've learned I can't appropriate His grace while responding to life in an unchristlike manner. So, I strive to "…stay always within the boundaries where God's love can reach and bless (me) you" (Jude 1:21, TLB). Once we begin to respond according to God's Word, we are then able to move on and clearly understand the choices we have to make.

I know you are struggling, even more than Mom and me, with a flood of emotions and it's difficult to think straight. I sense that this pregnancy represents the loss of everything you were holding dear. And, while it may appear to be that way on the surface, you have not lost everything when you have God as your Savior and Friend. In fact, by properly responding to God and His Word, you will gain far more than you ever imagined.

Remember, Amy, you have sought God's forgiveness and that means your slate is clean — as far as God is concerned you've committed no sin, ever! Mom and I, too, have forgiven you. We can walk down the street with our daughter as proud as we've ever been….

But what about the rest of your life? You have many difficult decisions to make. You have your life and the life of your baby to consider. There are no "perfect" answers…. I can't tell you what to do. You have engaged in an adult act and you have an adult decision to make. However, I want to point you to the context in which to make your decision. When you consider your options, do so with one central purpose in mind: "What will bring the most honor to God?"

Right choices will become clear as you (1) Maintain right attitudes (align yourself with God's Word during trying times, love those who mistreat you, and accept your humbling position with grace) (2) continue to consider only those options that would bring honor to God; and (3) Obtain wise counsel from mature Christians to confirm the leading you have.

If you decide to keep the baby, you can rest assured we will do all in our power to be the best grandparents possible. We will fill our responsibility in being a godly influence as best we can under God.

If you decide to relinquish the baby for adoption, you can rest assured we will be there to support you, love you, weep with you, and heal together with you.

I love you dearly, Amy, more than you can know. You will always be my little girl. There are brighter and more beautiful days ahead for all of us. God will use this as a stepping stone in all our lives. We will learn much together. We can more effectively minister to others because of how we allow God to use this in our lives.

Through this we can all become even closer as a family than before. Mom and I really felt honored and want to thank you for sharing this with us on the very day you found out. We thank you for the opportunity to be a part of the decisions that affect the life of our first grandchild. No matter what, this will always be a special child to both of us and we have lots of love to share with you and your first child – in whatever way God chooses to let us be a part.

The road may seem dark and lonely at times, but remember we're always here and want to help. And more importantly, Christ is with you always, your dearest Friend, your closest companion, the One who knows you most and loves you best. Mom and I pray for you daily. I love you, I love you, I love you.

Your Dad

Not a whole lot needs to be said after reading a letter like this one. Unfortunately, not every parent who has faced a similar situation has showed this much love and grace to their daughter. However, this letter teaches us all much about the unconditional love of a father who has committed his expectations, feelings, and his daughter's future to the Lord.

##  Take Action

The goal of this section has been to inform you about your teen's sexuality and to enlighten you as to your teen's sexual convictions (or, lack of them). Use the following Action Steps according to your own individual situation.

❏ After reading this section, would you and your spouse like to discuss certain items with your teen in more depth? If so, please list them below:

- _____
- _____
- _____

❏ Do you feel that you need to discuss your sexual boundaries and dating standards with your teen to help him define his own? Yes / No / I don't know

❏ Do you plan on communicating with your teen not only about the dangers of premarital sex but the joy, beauty, and fulfillment of sex in marriage?
Yes / No / I don't know

❏ Do you plan on talking with your spouse about being more affectionate with each other in front of the children? Yes / No / I don't know

❏ Do you want to help your teen avoid sexually compromising situations? If so, the following are a few suggestions:

- Never do anything that will violate your conscience (even for a person you really like when that person is probably using guilt to manipulate you into compromise).

- Abstain from all activity that causes sexual arousal. If holding hands causes you to get sexually aroused, then don't do it.

- Don't engage in petting (touching breasts and genitals) either inside or outside of one's clothing.

- If your relationship is frequently having problems with too much physical involvement, you may have to break it off in order to avoid going all the way.

- Set clear sexual and dating standards for yourself before you find yourself in a compromising situation.

- Don't compare your standards with your friend's standards especially if theirs seem to be lower than yours. God will honor your standards. Stick to the ones that are consistent with your conscience.

- Learn how to control your thought life. Avoid all sexual fantasizing.

- Always stand up for what you think is right whether your friends do or not.

- Control your emotions. When you get overly emotionally excited about someone, realize that it's probably just infatuation and talk your feelings through with someone who can help you gain perspective.

- Avoid all pornography, erotic literature, sexually explicit movies, and borderline romance novels.

❏ Plan on obtaining more information from your pastor or counselor about the teen "ring ceremony." This is for both a teenage son or daughter. The basic idea is that when your teen turns fifteen (or so) you buy him any ring that he wants as a symbol that he has made a special commitment to God, to himself, and to you to be morally pure and stay a virgin before marriage. On the evening of the ring presentation, you will take your teen out on a date (with full dinner), give him/her the special piece of jewelry, and talk about what his commitment to purity means. (Let your teen choose the piece of jewelry and the restaurant so that it will be something that he/she really likes.)

❏ After reading this section, have you come to realize that your own view of sex needs to change? Do you want to change your own perspective so that you can better educate your own teenager?

❏ Read a book and/or watch a video specifically designed for adolescents with your teenager. (*see the section Further Resources*).

# *5* **Pause to Reflect**

After doing the Action Steps that you feel fit your teen's needs, evaluate their effectiveness by answering the following questions so that you can learn to improve your communication.

● After talking with your teen, do you feel that he/she has a good understanding of the volatileness of natural sexual response and the necessity for standards of moral purity? Yes / No / I don't know

● How well did you "connect" with your teen in this section?
   Not very well    Unsure    Average    Very well

● How well did the Conversation Starters in this chapter work with your teen?
   Not very well    Average    Had problems with them    Very well

● What did you learn about your teen that you did not know before reading this section?

● What did you learn about yourself that you didn't know before reading this section?

● What did you learn about the other children in your family as a result of this information?

- What was your spouse's involvement with your teen in this section? Do you think that it could have been better? If so, in what way?

- Do you want to talk with someone rather urgently about your teen's sexual behavior or views? If so, with whom do you want to talk?

  _____
  _____
  _____

- Do you feel that your teen has the moral character to make right decisions concerning sexual activity? What makes you believe this?

- Record any further insights, questions, or comments concerning sex, morality, and your teen here:

## Further Resources

*The Missing Piece, Finding God's Peace For Your Past*, Lee Ezell, Harvest House, 1986.

*From One Single Mother to Another*, Sandra P. Aldrich, Regal Books, 1991.

*Daddy, I'm Pregnant*, "Bill", Multnomah Press, 1987.

*How To Help Your Child Say "NO" To Sexual Pressure*, Josh McDowell, Word Publishing, 1987.

Call: Your local Crisis Pregnancy Center for more information and counseling.

# CHAPTER TWENTY

# Mixed Messages: Forming Proper Sexual Identity

*I heard a story the other day of a little boy and girl who had just been introduced. They were trying to decide what games to play, and the little boy said, "I have an idea, let's play baseball."*

*But the little girl said, "Oh, no, I wouldn't want to do that; baseball is a boy's game. It's not feminine to run around on a dusty vacant lot. No, I wouldn't want to play baseball."*

*So the boy replied, "Okay, then, let's play football."*

*She answered, "Oh no, I wouldn't want to play football. That's even less feminine. I might fall and get dirty. No, that's not a girl's game."*

*He said, "Okay, I've got an idea. I'll race you to the corner."*

*She replied, "No, girls play quiet games; we don't run and get all sweaty. Girls should never race with boys."*

*The boy then scratched his head, trying to think of what she might want to do, and finally he said, "Okay, then let's play house."*

*She said, "Good! I'll be the daddy!"*[68]

Our society is filled with mixed messages about sexual identity. Humorous movies portray men dressing like women and women dressing like men. Television shows make fathers look dumb and wimpy. There are "unisex" salons and "unisex" clothes. Our teen's sexual identity is critically important. With all of the mixed gender messages being broadcast in our society today, how can we ensure that our teen will grow up without any gender confusion?

## 1 Know the Causes

During adolescence, teenagers feel many intense emotions. One of their greatest emotional needs is for unconditional love and acceptance. Like all of us, teens have a "love tank" deep inside of themselves. It's the place where they hold all of the love, attention, and affection that they receive from God and others. I have observed that during their adolescent years, teens have a leak in their "love tank." They need continual encouragement and care because they're still in the process of forming their own self-identity, which, when properly formed, will help them internally to know what to do to patch up their "love tank" any time they feel it leaking. But right now, they are too vulnerable and still "in the making," and, thus, they are not able to fill or repair their own tanks. They need the continual love of you and I to keep their tanks filled.

As you read the following list, see if your teen has "attached" himself to someone or something outside of God and the home that he may be using to fill up his leaking "love tank." By this list, I don't mean to say that I think that all of the following items are wrong or unhealthy. I just want to make you reflect upon the degree of emotional attachment that your son or daughter has put in any one direction and possibly the reasons why.

## 2 Observe Your Teen

Does your teen have an imbalanced or unnatural relationship with:

- someone of the opposite sex?

- a community/athletic club or a school/neighborhood gang?

- any time-consuming extracurricular activities, e.g., sports, choir, speech/debate, newspaper, yearbook, rally, etc.?

- a hobby which gives him a feeling of great pride and accomplishment?

- a horse, dog, bird, cat, etc. that provides him with deep emotional comfort?

- a same-sex best friend with whom he spends most of his time?

- a teacher, coach, youth leader, pastor, counselor, neighbor, or other adult?

Most parents would agree with me that most of the groups/activities listed above are not bad in themselves. However, it would be well worth it for you to ask yourself why your teen is so emotionally involved in a particular group or activity. Is it just for fun? Is it just because he's enjoying the development of his own natural talents? Or, is he lonely, confused, and in need of deep love and attention? Is he seeking in this person or activity to find his sexual/gender identity? This can be indicated by either your son or your daughter emotionally attaching him/herself to either a male or a "male" activity/group, or to a female or a "female" activity/group. What he emotionally "identifies with" all depends on his unmet emotional needs.

When you observe your teen getting "out of balance" in any area, a yellow flag should go up. Because every teen's life, personality, calling, talents, and interests are different, you shouldn't put your teen in a box or constantly compare him with others at school or church. However, use your own good judgment in assessing whether your teen has become imbalanced or extreme in a certain area by asking yourself whether he exhibits any potential signs of imbalance:

- an obsessive emotional attachment to someone/something; a misguided loyalty

- an immediate defensive reaction when questioned about it

- a totally closed mind; unwilling to talk or reason about it

- an over-commitment of time and schedule; duties and responsibilities are neglected

- a neglect of personal health, hygiene

- a constant fantasizing about it

- a compulsive talking about it

- it becomes the central, all-consuming focus of life/attention; nothing else matters

- becomes very secretive and protective about it

Parents of teens should monitor very closely what goes on in their teen's lives. This close attention is not to squelch their individuality or control their lives; it's to protect their emotional vulnerabilities and their sources of potential sexual identification. Be involved in your teen's activities. Go to all of their games or concerts. Watch their friends. Several teens shared with me that they were concerned about themselves because they felt close to a person of their same sex. "Does this mean I'm gay?," they asked me. In my response to their concern, I did not make light of their question. I asked them a few questions about their feelings toward the other person just to make sure that someone wasn't trying to entrap them. I then explained that it was very normal for them to have friends of the same sex with whom they felt very close. It's perfectly normal for teens, who are in the process of forming their sexual identities, to feel emotionally close to same-sex friends. It's also normal for teens to have thoughts of the same sex. But this does not mean that they are homosexual!

Do you remember what it was like being a teenager? It was tough, wasn't it? Teenagers are experiencing much more heartache on a more serious level than teens did a generation ago. Teenager's emotions are on a roller coaster ride much of the time. Any sense of security or belonging tends to bring a needed stability to their life. This is why parents should pay extra attention to the source which their teens are using to meet their emotional needs. If you do believe that your child is involved in a dangerous situation: a gang, a boy/girlfriend relationship that you cannot put a stop to, or a homosexual relationship, please get professional Christian help immediately.

The number of teens becoming gay is heart-rending. Without good relationships with their fathers, in need of male attention and bonding, many teens are selling themselves on the streets in an effort to meet their emotional need for Dad. Recently, I spoke with one of the members of the task force appointed by our governor to see what could be done about the male teen prostitutes in the city in which I live. This task force member told me that there were approximately 2,000 teen male prostitutes on the streets in our city. Many of them have been kicked out of their own homes. Teen gender identity is of crucial importance.

People learn from their own experiences. Because of my experiences as a teen-ager and from my observation of young girls, I have a deep concern for the unhealthy emotional attachments that young girls as well as young boys can find themselves entrapped. It is my observation that the unhealthy relationship may begin very purely and innocently. What might seem like a good friendship with an individual may turn sour as the adult or stronger influence takes unfair advantage of the trust and emotional bonding.

This outside influence that can change the life of a young person forever may come in from many avenues. A neighbor may give a lonely teen special and needed attention. A member of the family may exert a controlling influence on the innocence of a girl or boy. A trusted teacher, coach, or other significant adult in the life of a vulnerable young person may take unfair advantage of the friendship.

This section is not intended to provoke fear. It is, however, intended to remind us all that we need to stay alert and keep a watch on our young people as they grow into maturity. Remember, Satan comes in sheep's clothing to steal, kill and destroy.

Even if you don't think that confusion over his/her sexual identity is a problem for your son or daughter, and even if you don't have any concern about an unhealthy relationship your teen may be having, read the following excerpt so that you will be more equipped to help a confused teen whenever the Lord may bring him/her across your path.

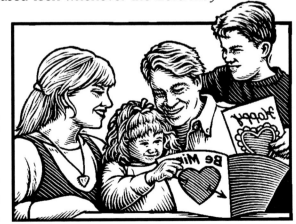

### Loving Parents: The Key to Gender Identity:

"The security we feel in our sense of maleness or femaleness seems to have a profound effect on our capacity to relate heterosexually. A major study conducted in 1981 concluded that in light of many variables, one consistent theme among the homosexuals studied was gender confusion…. Adult homosexuals recall a sense of being different from their same-sex peer group in childhood. That gender confusion is paired later in life with an erotic preference for the same sex…. That study has theological implications as well as sexual ones. Genesis 1:27 claims that God created humanity to reflect His image in duo form — as male and female. ["And God created man in His own image, in the image of God He created him; male and female He created them."] Implicit here is the need for each human creature to secure a sufficiently clear sense of gender. Then, as either male or female, we can seek a needed counterpart in the opposite sex…. [But what contributes to gender confusion in the first place?] One cannot de-emphasize the powerful role parents play in a child's acquisition of gender identity. Mom and Dad are our first and most influential models of what a man and woman are and help determine what characteristics we will internalize that are appropriate to our gender….

Perhaps the most powerful influence on our gender comes from [our relationship with our same-sex parent]. Through the parent of the same sex, we gain, or do not gain, a needed resource of identification and intimacy that we incorporate as part of our own maleness or femaleness…. An affirming relationship with the same-sex parent proves affirming to one's gender. Breaches in relationship with the same-sex parent (e.g., parent's abuse, personal victimization, emotional detachment, death, illness, neglect, etc.) can block the lifeline of intimacy and identification which in turn obstructs a child's secure gender development….

[The opposite-sex parent also] plays a vital role in affirming, or not affirming, the child's gender, in that he/she encounters the child as the other sex, a relationship which will influence future means of relating to the opposite sex. The opposite-sex parent is intended to convey our adequacy, even our goodness as a person of the opposite gender….

The result of gender confusion is often loneliness and fear, with a distrust of our capacity to operate successfully out of our respective genders. We may have come to doubt our ability to relate well to our own sex, while the opposite sex may have become a primary point of identification. Not fitting in, we may have come to fear our sexuality — our gender, our bodies, ourselves. [Thus,] homosexual love is not a genuine sexual preference. It's more of a striving to complete one's own unmet needs for same-sex intimacy and identification."

### *Our Loving Heavenly Father: The Key to Healing Gender Confusion:*

"[We must remember that] fallen self cannot know itself. In other words, the creature cannot truly discover himself through another creature or thing. [In a teen's striving for self-identity] homosexuality is one expression of seeking an identity outside of the Creator (Romans 1:18–32). True self-knowledge comes from outside ourselves, as the Creator tells us who we are. That necessitates an openness on our part to a new self-definition. The Creator must name us, His created, according to His original intent — heterosexuality…. Identifying oneself in terms of homosexuality may be clinically unsound. Leanne Payne writes that: There is really no such thing as a "homosexual" person. There are only those who need healing of old rejections and deprivations, deliverance from the wrong kind of self-love and the actions that issue from it, and — along with that — the knowledge of their own higher selves in Christ…."

[The following is an excellent prayer for a new sexual identity in Christ:] "Father, we come to you now and want to lay at the feet of Your Son, Jesus, the Crucified One, any word, any label, any way in which we define ourselves that runs contrary to who we really are in Christ… We identify and lay down the label of homosexual. We take authority over that lie, that label that defined us falsely for too long…. Now, with resurrection authority, we receive the true words You give to us, Father. We receive the blessed realities that we are Your sons and daughters, and that You have freed us to accept our true heterosexual identities. Give us Your true words of self-definition. We give You, our Creator, the full right to define us. You have made us; now name us."[69]

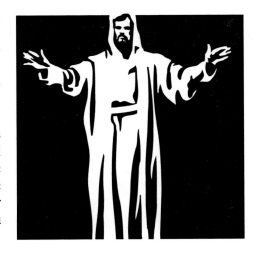

Your teen may have never thought of the deep despair that lies within the heart of a homosexual. He/she may feel a sense of disgust whenever the subject of homosexuality is addressed in the news or other source. We can teach our teens that the love of the Father is for all man[woman]kind. Although the lifestyle of a homosexual is sinful, God hates the sin but loves the sinner. It is my prayer that Christians can portray the love of God and the power of prayer for wholeness for those whose lives have been broken by sexual sin and immorality. In my early Christian walk, those who discipled me always reminded me that "we are the only Bible that some will ever read, we are the only Christ that some will ever see...."

The following are a few suggestions to help start a conversation concerning this delicate issue.

## 3 Talk with Your Teen

After reading all of the following questions, choose which ones would be the most effective ways for you to use to begin a casual conversation with your teen. Remember that your purpose is to get your teen to open up — not shut down as a result of you dominating the conversation.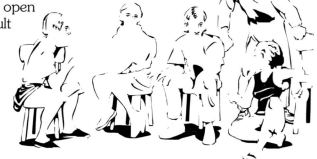

- *"What do you feel/think when you hear about or see a person who is a homosexual?"*

- *"If someone close to you (brother/sister/relative) were gay, would that change the way you thought of homosexuals?"*

- *"If Jesus were to walk down the street and meet a homosexual, what do you think His response would be?"*

- *"Why do you think a person becomes gay?"*

- *"Do you think that being a homosexual is inherent at birth or is learned?"*

- *"What do you think is the major contributing factor to an individual becoming a homosexual? Why?"*

- *"Do you think that a homosexual can ever be changed (healed) and thus have a normal, happy marital relationship with the opposite sex?"*

- *"Have you ever talked to your friends about this issue?" "If so, what have they said about it?"*

- *"If a homosexual visited your youth group at church, became a Christian and shared his/her testimony, how would you feel about hanging around or being friends with that person?"*

# 4 Take Action

The goal of this section is to heighten your awareness of the sexual identity issues that face teenagers today. Do not be alarmed at the information. I hope you have no use for it with your own teen; however, if you ever encounter one who needs to know the way to healing of an unnatural affection, the information in this section would be helpful.

❏ Go to a Christian bookstore together and find an autobiography or biography of a homosexual. Read it together to gain insight into the real struggles of the gay lifestyle. (Use wisdom in your selection). The goal is to develop more of a heart of compassion rather than disgust.

❏ If you are concerned about your teen and his/her relationship with a person of the same sex, be very careful but try to engage your teen in a conversation about that friendship. Your son or daughter may be just waiting for someone to reach out and notice the situation and give him/her help.

❏ In any case, whenever discussing the homosexual lifestyle, the conversation should be a balanced one of God's true feelings against the sin of homosexuality and the mercy of God's unconditional love for the individual. Although it makes Him angry to see lives destroyed by such a lifestyle, His heart is grieved for the individuals involved.

❏ Find a professional Christian counselor who specializes in counseling the homosexual. Make sure you interview the person and find out if he/she believes that a gay person can/should change to a heterosexual life.

❏ After reading this section, do you feel that your son or daughter has a healthy view of his/her sexual identity?   Yes   No   How do I find out?

❏ If you are uncertain about your teenager's position on his/her sexuality, seek professional help. You may try to talk to him/her about how they feel about marriage and intimacy with the opposite sex, but be careful that your teen doesn't become defensive or conclude that he/she is a homosexual.

# *5* **Pause to Reflect**

After doing the Action Steps appropriate for your situation, evaluate the "connection" you made with your teen.

- After talking with my teenager about this subject, how confident are you that he has a positive view of the opposite sex/the same sex?

  Not confident        Somewhat confident        Very confident

- How well did you "connect" with your teen on the subject of sexual identity?

  Not very successfully        Somewhat successfully        Very successfully

- How well did the Conversation Starters in this section work for you?

  Not very well        Fairly well        Very well

- What have you learned about your teen that you may not have known before reading this section?

- What have you learned about homosexuality that you may not have known before reading this section?

- What is your spouse's opinion concerning this subject?

- Record any further insights, questions, or comments concerning your teen and his/her sexual identity here:

# Further Resources

*Someone I Love is Gay, How Family and Friends Can Respond*, Anita Worthen & Bob Davies, Intervarsity Press, 1996.

*Setting Love in Order: Hope and Healing for the Homosexual*, Mario Bergner, Baker Books, 1995.

*Pursuing Sexual Wholeness: How Jesus Heals the Homosexual*, Andrew Comiskey, Creation House, 1989.

*The Broken Image*, Leanne Payne, Crossway Books, 1981.

*Coming Out of Homosexuality*, Bob Davies and Lori Rentzel, Intervarsity Press, 1993.

# CHAPTER TWENTY-ONE

# The Dating Game

While a youth pastor was preaching to his youth group one evening, he noticed a young teenager with his arm around his girlfriend. The youth pastor had known that these two teenagers had been dating for awhile. He then noticed this young man lean over and give his girlfriend a kiss. After the meeting, the youth pastor walked up to the young man and asked, "Do you plan on marrying this young lady?" Startled that the youth pastor would ask such a question, he answered, "Well, no, of course not!" And the pastor replied, "Then, why are you kissing another man's wife?"

By now, I'm sure, the subject of dating has been a hot topic in your home. As I talked to my students about dating, all they could talk about was how much fun they were missing if they weren't allowed to date. If their parents had postponed their freedom to date until they reached a certain age, they could hardly wait to celebrate the arrival of that day!

## 1 Know the Causes

The time for dating can be an exciting and fun time, but it can also be a time of heartache and depression. I always ruined my students' eager anticipation to date whenever I shared with them this simple fact: Dating isn't always fun! I would like to talk to the people who invented dating. I would like to share with them all of the unnecessary pain and hurt that I experienced throughout high school when I single-dated: feeling the rejection when a guy I liked asked me out only once and then never talked to me again; feeling the confusion when other more "popular" girls seemed to have such a blast on a date and I could not relate; feeling the rejection when only the "unpopular" boys asked me out; feeling the guilt when I hurt a guy's feelings or went along with something I knew was not right. This on and off emotional roller coaster could have been too much for me if it weren't for my extracurricular activities that conveniently kept me too busy to date.

It wasn't until my freshman year in college that all of my emotional bumps and bruises motivated me enough to decide I had better adopt some concrete dating standards. During high school, I couldn't blame all of my dating grief on my parents. After all, my grandparents had never taught my parents any specific dating standards either.

## 2 Observe Your Teen

Unfortunately, most teens don't have any dating standards whatsoever. Even in Christian circles, controversy and differing opinions are obvious. The following questions will help you discover whether or not your teen has developed any dating principles. Your teen's responses to these queries will also help you to find out how open he/she is to forming some standards.

- Have you and your teen ever discussed the issue of dating?

  Yes    No    I don't remember    Planning on it soon

- What have you and your teen decided about the question of single-dating?

  Believe in it    Don't believe in it    Don't believe in it until a certain age    Still undecided

- What have you and your teen decided about the practice of group-dating?

  Believe in it    Don't believe in it    Don't believe in it until a certain age    Still undecided

- What have you and your teen decided about the practice of formal courtship?

  Believe in it    Don't believe in it    Don't believe in it until a certain age    Still undecided

- We have decided together with our teen that he/she will not be allowed to single-date until the age of:

  13–14 years old    15–16 years old    17–18 years old    19 years +

- If your teen hasn't formed any of his own dating standards, does he understand, and has he willingly agreed to live by yours?

  Yes    No    I don't know    Will discuss it soon.

- As parents, do you plan to be very involved in your teenager's dating life?

  Yes / No / I don't know

- After dating someone five or six times, your teen knows that your standard for physical involvement is what?
  - ❑ no physical touching
  - ❑ holding hands only
  - ❑ hugs only
  - ❑ short kisses on the cheek
  - ❑ kissing and hugging OK
  - ❑ no French kissing
  - ❑ no petting

## Dating Standards

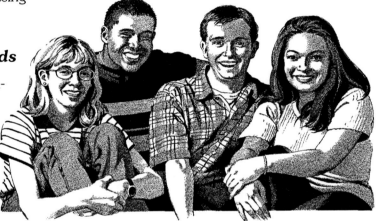

There are many reasons why dating is not always fun for teens. There are many causes which combine to make it sometimes very painful and disappointing for them. Some of these causes are: emotional vulnerability, experiential naiveté, undeveloped common sense, lack of parental instruction and/or involvement, and a lack of dating standards. A lack of dating standards includes a lack in having a standard concerning who to date as well as a lack in the sexual and social behavior acceptable on the date.

Because of the potential problems with single-dating, you and your teen must decide what your teen's personal dating standards will be. Each Christian family is different, and each family has its own convictions based on their fundamental values and world view. If you and your teen have already set guidelines concerning dating, congrats! If not, don't back down from forming them clearly and concisely even when the pressure or opposition seems intense. Without judging any other parent's dating standards or beliefs, I think that most would agree with me that Satan enjoys throwing two unprepared teens all alone into an emotionally and sexually explosive context and see them struggle and fail. The heart of the devil is to destroy your teen's purity and innocence any way that he can. He knows by experience that if he can seriously ensnare innocent Christian teens in the works of the flesh, add emotional confusion, frustration, guilt, and secrecy on top of it, that it's possible for him to damage the families of the ensuing generations.

Therefore, it's essential that even if your teen isn't very open to forming dating standards at this time, that you work the hardest at maintaining open lines of communication about the subject in general. If you have not already made your decision about dating and dating standards, it's not too late. It wasn't until I graduated from high school that I developed some firm dating standards. "Better late than never!"

## *General Dating Guidelines*

If you and your teen haven't formed any dating standards as yet, or if you want some fresh input, you can use the ideas in this next section to stimulate discussion.

- **Make specific plans for any dating activity.** Whether your teen is going out on a single-date or a group date, it's important to plan the time well. "If you fail to plan, you plan [for your teen] to fail." Teens will not do well in a dating context if they are allowed to just "hang around just to see what happens." Know exactly where they are going, with whom they are going, what they are going to do there, and when they will return. Hear your teen verbalize his commitments to you and hold him/her to them. Non-accusingly and with kindness and patience, question them about any inconsistencies.

- **Be Creative.** Have fun together with your teen listing many fun, dating ideas. Some will be common ideas, but others will be highly creative. Others will be impressed because you came up with such unique activities. See the suggestions on page 362 in the *Total Health* student text.

- **Train your teen about God's order for successful relationships.** When discussing dating, there's a tendency to jump right into a discussion

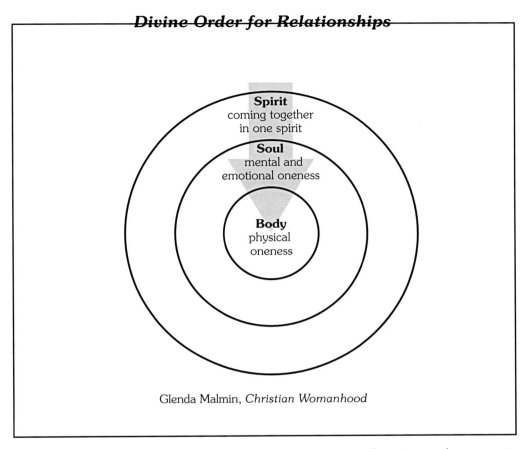

**Spirit**
coming together
in one spirit

**Soul**
mental and
emotional oneness

**Body**
physical
oneness

Glenda Malmin, *Christian Womanhood*

on the sexual aspect of the relationship because moral purity is what parents are concerned with the most. Explain to your teen why God's order for successful relationships is the successful model to follow. Demonstrate to him how it will protect him emotionally and sexually. Make clear to him how it will lead him into a satisfying, long-term relationship; just what he desires deep inside. God's order is: first bond in spirit (through love of God, prayer, Bible, witnessing, church, worship, values, ministries) then bond in soul (intellectually, emotionally, volitionally, directionally, and practically), and lastly, bond in body (sexual arousal and intercourse in marriage). Many teens reverse this order and experience drastic consequences.

When teens begin to date, their immediate temptation is to reverse God's order and to begin with sexually arousing physical involvement. One reason that this happens so commonly is because expressing physical affection is the easiest and quickest way to "communicate" acceptance and specialness. The result, however, is an unhealthy emotional and physical bond that produces guilt and frustration. Getting to know someone spiritually, intellectually, and emotionally first takes more time, is harder work, and is a slower process. But, because it's God's way, it's safer, happier, and pays lifelong dividends. You can use the high divorce statistics in our nation to help you to make this point.

- **Keep involved.** Never give up with your teen. Although he's naturally becoming more independent all the time, don't quit being involved. Your teen needs you now even though it seems he's pushing you away. The key to your continuing success with your teen is finding the right way to stay involved in his life. The following are some ideas about how you can be involved in your teen's dating life:

  ❏ Interview your teen's dates before you give them permission to go out.

  ❏ Ask questions about where they're going, what they plan to do, and when they will return (not when they plan to return).

  ❏ When they return, ask them what they did, and where they went. (See if they did exactly what they said they were going to do).

  ❏ Have a specific time to for them to come back.

  ❏ Have dates at your home doing family things, i.e., game night, movie night, special dinner/BBQ, sporting activities.

  ❏ Meet the parents of the person your teen wants to date before they go out. Do more than chat with them over the phone. How do they impress you?

  ❏ With a humble attitude, share your dating standards and expectations with the person your teen is dating as well as his/her parents.

- **Create a desire in your teen for kingdom relationships.** Today's culture promotes a life philosophy of "me-first." Self-interest controls everyone who is not following Jesus. The seeds of this mentality trickle down into the most important relationship between two people — marriage. Pastor Wendell Smith put it this way: "Don't use the world's way to relate... or you'll get the world's results."[70] The following chart shows the difference between the dating culture in America and the dating culture in God's kingdom.[71] Which dating culture do you think has influenced your teen the most up to this point?

| God's Ways of "Kingdom Relationships" <br> *God-centered relationships* | | Culture's Way of "Dating": <br> *Self-centered relationships* | |
|---|---|---|---|
| **Basis:** | Wholesome attraction <br> Commitment to God <br> Friendship | **Basis:** | Natural attraction <br> Feelings, desires |
| **Goal:** | Mutual edification and <br>     fulfillment of God's will | **Goal:** | Mutual gratification and <br>     fulfillment of self-will |
| **Qualities:** | Giving attitude <br> Absolute moral standards <br> Focus on Spirit and Soul <br> Taking time to get to know each <br>     other <br> Relationship inclusive of the <br>     Body of Christ | **Qualities:** | Receiving attitude <br> No absolutes, no standards <br> Focus on Body and Soul <br> Moving quickly to take <br>     advantage of each other <br> Relationship exculsive and <br>     possessive |
| **Results:** | Stronger relationship to the Lord <br>     and others <br> Healthy self-image <br> Character development for better <br> Greater motivation <br> Increased fulfillment <br> Good example to others <br> Peace, joy and abundant life | **Results:** | Weakened relationships <br>     with God and others <br> Unhealthy self-image <br> Character change for worse <br> Draining of motivation <br> Decreased fulfillment <br> Influence others to sin <br> Confusion, strife and heartache <br> Emptiness and sorrow |

Iverson, Smith, Scheidler, Malmin, *Confronting Our Culture*

- **Be open to the alternatives to traditional single-dating.** There are other alternatives to the traditional dating models in our society. In line with its own convictions, each family needs to discover what works in their home. It's possible for teenagers to still have fun without the social and sexual pressures that come with dating. When your teen chooses not to single-date (i.e., go out with one person alone on a consistent basis), then he can spend more time focusing on academics, school activities, family, friends, his relationship with the Lord, and the development of special talents and interests.

- **Before you look at some viable alternatives to single-dating, you need to ask yourself what the purpose of single-dating really is.** Some parents may disagree on the answer, but it's essential for parents to come to an understanding of what they see is the reason for single-dating before they decide whether they want to allow or encourage their son or daughter to become involved in it. The closer that parents come to viewing the true purpose of single-dating, the more they will be able to evaluate its fruit in their own teenager's life. There are some parents who begin to allow their teen to single-date, but after seeing certain results with their son or daughter, change their minds.

Very specifically, and most importantly, what is the real purpose of single-dating? More generally, and somewhat less importantly, why do teens single-date? Do they single-date to have fun, to get to know someone better, to learn how to have positive male/female relationships, or because pressure from their peers and society pushes them into it? All of these options reflect the facts of a teen's social reality in some way, but, I believe, there's one main reason for formal, single-dating that is often overlooked: to pursue a marriage partner.

Some parents may disagree with me on this, but I feel that the main reason why some parents would not accept the idea that the main purpose would probably be because they have adopted the American culture's commercial emphasis upon teens having "fun" rather than seeing more closely what really happens when teens single-date. I also agree with the statement that dating prepares young people for divorce. They learn how to "break up" rather than how to be committed.

All of us have to admit, I think, that our own dating experiences when we were teens affect how we come to view single-dating for our teens. If we happened to have had an overall good experience, then we would probably be more favorable to the idea than if we had an overall bad teen dating experience. In deciding what is best for your teen now, try not only to be as objective as possible, but open to what is the best spiritual and moral good for your teen. Individual teen maturity levels also would play into your decision. Either way, if you're interested in exploring some other alternatives to traditional single-dating, here are a few very workable ideas:

**Group Activity:** Teens can really have a lot of fun and still get to know each other as individuals in group activities. There are many different kinds of groups that your teen can become a part of, e.g., church, youth, YMCA, YWCA, Boy Scouts, Girl Scouts, 4H, local sports leagues, neighborhood, ad hoc committees, community service, charities, school field trips, band, choir, speech/debate, school newspaper, equestrians, school yearbook, photography club, chess club, etc. All of these provide your teen the benefit of having other people around. This greatly decreases the social and sexual pressures inherent in single-dating.

**Group-Dating:** Group dating is going out with several friends. There may be couples in the group, but not necessarily. The group can be comprised of an even or odd number. If you want to, you may even invite a chaperone to join the group. The following are some good reasons why I think that group-dating is a good alternative to single-dating:

- It empowers a teenager to get to know members of the opposite sex without pressure.

- It sanctions a teenager to observe how his/her friends respond in different settings.

- It allows a teenager the safety of numbers.

- It encourages a teenager to get to know someone first on a casual, informal basis.

**Double/Triple-Dating:** A double or triple date is simply several couples going out together. The benefit here is safety of numbers, but the danger is that each couple may pair off by themselves to become romantically or sexually involved. In my view, the double or triple date would be preferable for older, more mature teens whom you can trust to be going out to have a fun time as a group and not primarily as "couples."

**Parent-Dating:** Parent-dating is going out either in a group, one couple, or several couples with Mom and Dad as a couple. This idea would seem odd to some, but for those who have a good relationship with their parents and whose parents are not overly-controlling, this idea could work great, especially for younger teens. E.g., everybody could drive to the mall together, split up into couples for a little while, and then come back together again. One of the prerequisites of this kind of dating practice, would be that Dad and Mom would have to be very loving yet very firm about their desire to be closely involved in their teen's dating life. If a boy wanted to date your daughter, he would have to prove his pure intentions by respecting Dad and Mom's way of him getting to know their daughter and them getting to know him!

**Courtship:** An old but new approach to getting to know a person. The parents and family are involved as a young man requests permission to court a young lady. Activities are focused around the family with open communication and mutual respect. This works if both families of the young people involved share the same conviction concerning courtship.

## 3 Talk with Your Teen

After reading all of the following questions, choose which ones would be the most effective ways for you to use to begin a casual conversation with your teen. Remember that your purpose is to get your teen to open up — not shut down as a result of you dominating the conversation.

- *"What do you expect from dating?"*

- *"What do you think is the purpose of single-dating?"*

- *"How do you feel about the standards we have concerning dating?"*

- *"Do you have any fears associated with dating?"*

- *"What are the sorts of activities that your date likes to do? Where does he/she like to go?"*

- *"What sorts of things does your date talk about with you while on a date?"* (If the answer is, "He/she doesn't talk much," you should ask what they do if they don't talk.)

- *"What are some excuses that you have heard your friends make to compromise their dating standards?"* (E.g., if they say that their standard is only to date growing Christians, but they like someone who is not a Christian, what is their reason for compromising this standard?)

- *"Why is it important not to have physical involvement in a relationship?"*

- *"Why do teenagers think that dating is fun? What makes single-dating fun?"*

- *"Do you have any friends who have been hurt by single-dating for awhile and then breaking up? Why do you think they got hurt? How does this make you feel?"*

- *"I have heard it said that single-dating just prepares a person for divorce later in life. What do you think that means and do you agree or disagree?"*

## 4 Take Action

The goal of this section is to help you and your teen make some firm dating standards. If you've already agreed on some clear dating guidelines, then the Conversation Starters and the Action Steps will reinforce what you've already decided. If you haven't, then the following steps will help you to do so:

❏ After reading this section and talking with your teen, do you feel that you already have a good set of dating standards for your teen?

Yes / No / I don't know

❏ After reading this section, do you feel that you and your spouse need to get together with your teen and draw up some specific dating standards?

Yes / No / I don't know

❏ After reading this section, do you feel that you need to get more involved in your teen's dating and social life? If so, how will you do this? List your plans below.

_____

_____

_____

❏ After reading this section, do you feel that your spouse needs to get more involved in your teen's dating and social life? If so, how will he/she do this? List your plans below.

_____

_____

_____

❏ Have your teen record the qualities he/she desires in a wife/husband. Then, discuss the need for him/her to develop the same qualities in him/herself.

❏ One of the dating standards that you and your spouse have discussed with your teen is that he/she will only date growing Christians.

Yes      No      Not yet decided

## 5 Pause to Reflect

After doing the Action Steps appropriate for your situation, improve the next "connection" with your teen by evaluating this last one.

● After talking with your teen about this material, how confident are you that he/she is prepared for the dating years? Yes / No / I don't know

● How well did you "connect" with your teen on the subject of dating?

Not very successfully      Somewhat successfully      Very successfully

● How well did this chapter's Conversation Starters work with your teen?

Not very well      Fairly well      Very well

● Do you feel confident that you don't need to consider making any changes in your teen's present dating standards? Yes / No / I don't know

- After reading this material and talking with your teen, how do you feel about single-dating and your teen?

- What is your spouse's opinion concerning single-dating and your teen?

- What did you learn about your teen that you didn't know before reading this section?

- Record any further insights, questions, or comments concerning your teen and dating here:

## Further Resources

*Of Knights and Fair Maidens* (pro-courting), Jeff and Danielle Myers, 1996.

*Hassles, Problems that Hit Home, 7 Sessions on Family and Dating*, Lyman Coleman, Serendipity House, 1994.

*Givers, Takers and Other Kinds of Lovers*, Josh McDowell, Tyndale House Publishers.

*The Love Killer,* Josh McDowell and Bob Hostetler, Word, Inc.

*Passion and Purity,* Elisabeth Elliot, Revell.

*Dating vs. Courtship*, Paul Jehle, Plymouth Rock Foundation, 1993.
For more information on courtship, contact:

The Courtship Connection
3731 Cecelia
Toledo, OH 43608
(419) 729–4594

# Tobacco, Alcohol, and Drugs

*Many Christian parents assume that church membership and involvement in youth ministry will produce spiritually mature youngsters. Active churchgoing parents are stunned to learn that their "good" children are dabbling in substance abuse...[72]*

Twenty years ago, teenagers worried about having the right clothes, getting a date for the dance, being on time for class, being respectful to the teachers, and, at worst, sneaking a beer or a cigarette. Today, teenagers are at risk from many different kinds of drugs, alcohol, crime, gangs, suicide, pornography, rape, and STDs including AIDS.

It's been said that, "Experience is the best teacher." But, is that really true? When applied to teens making serious mistakes in their lives, the belief would say that the best way for a teen to learn to do right is by making many mistakes and then learning from them. Personally, I would like my children to learn from the bad experiences and misjudgments of others rather than from the scars of their own wrong choices. Ron Mehl, senior pastor of Beaverton Foursquare Church, calls learning from others' mistakes, "guided experiences." If your teen was to hear a stranger share his painful experience with trying to quit drinking alcohol, would it be enough to keep your teen from taking a drink? If your teen had a close friend whose father died of alcohol related illness would your teen be more likely to pay attention? Unfortunately in most cases, for teens to change their behavior from hearing about others' predicaments, the painful consequences have to be very close to their own lives to carry such an impact.

# *1* **Know the Causes**

For the teenagers who are abnormally curious and who have not formed a strong personal conviction against tobacco, alcohol, or drugs, someone's testimony wouldn't be enough to keep them from trying it. Why? Because most teens feel as if they are indestructible. They think that their life will be totally different than the person who had the big problem. They don't see the possibility of the worst also happening to them. Teens are notorious for not looking past the weekend. They don't grasp the fact that the choices they make today will definitely affect their future. What teen who starts to drink plans on becoming an alcoholic who can't keep a job or his marriage? What teen who smokes marijuana plans on becoming a cocaine addict who dies of an overdose?

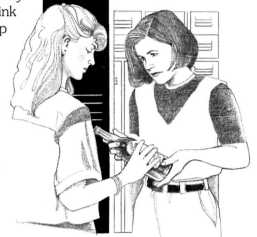

The unwise choice of most teens to experiment with addictive substances is due to the following five factors: curiosity, peer pressure (desiring to feel accepted by fitting in with the group), seeking to fill their "love tank" in some way, escaping the pain of their lives, and experimentation. Keeping these factors in mind, it is important that parents keep alert for any sign that could warn them of their teenager's dangerous dabblings.

What else causes Christian teenagers to experiment with drugs, alcohol, or tobacco? Benny and Sheree Phillips list the following as some of the reasons why Christian teens may succumb to these unhealthy and addictive influences.[73]

- **A Faulty Spiritual Foundation:** Parents impassioned about their relationship with Jesus Christ will infect their children with zeal for God and His Church. Jesus did not call us to follow a church building or church program, He said to follow Him, the person of Jesus Christ. Young people respond to challenges, not rituals; people not institutions. An authentic Christian lifestyle is our most effective tool to create in our children a distaste for all that the world can offer them.

- **Misguided Priorities:** One of the major consequences of living in a fast-paced, materialistic culture is a loss of time with our children; a lack of quality family time. Time is a precious resource. It's tragic if wasted, priceless if well-invested. Our children's very futures, even their spiritual development, may be greatly determined by how we use the few years we have to train, love, and build wholesome memories into them.

- **A False Definition of Spirituality:** Christian teenagers who have been around "spiritual" Christians long enough know the act. Parents must be careful not to judge their teen's spiritual health merely by externals, i.e., how frequently their teen brings up spiritual issues, how they seem to enjoy going to church or youth meetings, how much they remember of the sermon, or even how impressively they worship God. These all have their place, but they must not be the sole measure of a teen's relationship to God. What's more critical is possessing genuine character behind all the religious actions.

- **Harmful Influences:** I don't think any Christian parent knowingly or willingly allows harmful influences into their children's lives. Harmful influences, however, don't always have immediate negative results. Have you ever noticed, for instance, how long it takes to rid your child's vocabulary of certain words he has heard only a few times in the neighborhood? Or, what about the lasting impression one soap opera love scene can leave on the minds of our young people? Protecting our children from harmful influences means that we need other people to be on the lookout with us; other Christian friends who might notice something that we miss. If your teenager attends a Christian school, it's vitally important that you see their Christian school and staff as a part of the help you need with your teen. Your teenager's teachers are an extra pair of eyes and ears for you. Do everything you can to work with them, not against them. If the school staff makes a mistake, which they are bound to do, kindly share your thoughts and pray that they have divine wisdom adequate for each decision.

## 2 Observe Your Teen

The following observations may help you discover the inner convictions your teen may have concerning the use of harmful substances.

- Of the four reasons previously given as to why teens may use harmful substances, in what category, if any, do you feel your teen may be weak?
  - ❑ A faulty spiritual foundation
  - ❑ Misguided priorities
  - ❑ A false definition of spirituality
  - ❑ Harmful influences

- Are you or your spouse concerned about your teen's basic Christian character or commitment? Yes / No / I don't know

- Do you think that your teen might be tempted to try tobacco, drugs, or alcohol? Yes / No / I don't know

- Do you think that any of your teenager's friends are a bad influence on him especially concerning harmful substances? What about the family members of your teen's friends? Yes / No / I don't know

- Has communication with your teen recently shut down? Yes / No / I don't know

- Does your teen seem secretive, spending much of his time alone?
  Yes / No / I don't know

- Does your teen avoid family gatherings and family activities?
  Yes / No / I don't know

- During normal conversation, does your teen frequently avoid eye contact with you, your spouse, and other family members? Yes / No / I don't know

- Is your teen passive and indifferent toward most things? Yes / No / I don't know

- When you've asked your teen about his possible use of drugs, alcohol, or tobacco, is his response always short and does he quickly change the subject?
  Yes / No / I don't know

- Have others voiced a concern about your teen having a real or potential substance abuse problem? Yes / No / I don't know

- Have you noticed the smell of smoke on your teenager's clothing?
  Yes / No / I don't know

- Have you found items in your teen's room that have led you to believe that he may be involved with drugs and/or alcohol? Yes / No / I don't know

  If so, list the items here:



- Have you noticed a change in your teen's appearance; a lack of personal hygiene or an odd clothing style? Yes / No / I don't know

- Is your teen's academic performance suffering? Yes / No / I don't know

- Have your teen's sleeping patterns changed? Yes / No / I don't know

- Has your teen been lying? Yes / No / I don't know

- Has your teen's behavior seemed erratic or unusual at times?
  Yes / No / I don't know

- Does your teen have a self-esteem lower than usual? Yes / No / I don't know

- Has your teen become unusually rude (sarcastically defensive) recently?
  Yes / No / I don't know

- Has your teen been skipping school or been consistently late to school lately?
  Yes / No / I don't know

- Does your teen go outside at odd times for no apparent reason?
  Yes / No / I don't know

- Do matches seem to be disappearing from your house?
  Yes / No / I don't know

- Has any money, in small or large amounts, been disappearing from your house? Yes / No / I don't know

- Has your teen been more argumentative lately? Yes / No / I don't know

- Has your teen been more absent-minded and forgetful recently?
  Yes / No / I don't know

- Have you noticed a change in your teen's eating habits? Yes / No / I don't know

- Has your teen been losing quite a bit of weight? Yes / No / I don't know

- Do your teen's eyes look lifeless? Yes / No / I don't know

- Has your teen been acting evasive? Yes / No / I don't know

- Has your teen all of a sudden started using eye drops or mints?
  Yes / No / I don't know

- Does your teen seem depressed much of the time? Yes / No / I don't know

If your answer to several of these observation questions is yes, then you may have reason to suspect your teen is involved with smoking, alcohol, or drugs. It's normal to try to find logical excuses for your teen's unusual behaviors and attitudes. Don't look at the individual signs. Look more at the unusual patterns.

## 3 Talk with Your Teen

Once teenagers have crossed over the line and involved themselves in a strong negative influence, the first thing that usually goes is communication. Teens significantly decrease their interactions with their parents through: being less available, cutting talks short, constantly having to go somewhere else, and being superficial and evasive. Teens cut off their dialogue with their parents, most probably, because they want to avoid exposure, confrontation, discipline, or potential restrictions. At the very time that communication is the most important, it becomes the most tenuous and delicate. Teens may refuse to respond to their parents. They may totally ignore their efforts at bridge-building. Worst, they may make fun of their parents and respond with goofy, silly answers.

The last thing teens want to feel is that they are being interrogated. If teens choose to answer their parent's questions openly and honestly, their parents should not act shocked or surprised, get angry, or lecture them on the spot. A thought to help parents in such a situation to help to control their anger is the thought: "At least my teen is getting this out in the open; now, maybe we can all do something about it!"

When teens use drugs, they usually lie about it. If you believe that your teen may have a substance abuse problem, don't believe him if he just answers, "I only tried it once" or, "I'll never do it again." Seek professional help, and try to do what the counselors ask you to do. At some point, confrontation must occur. Be strong. Face the reality. Things may get worse before they get better. Without a doubt, however, you cannot afford to ignore or rationalize the problem. Thinking, "This is only a phase," or "She will get over it," will only bring disastrous results. Also, if you have been rescuing your teen from the consequences of his/her own poor choices, stop.

After reading all of the following questions, choose which ones would be the most effective ways for you to use to begin a casual conversation with your teen. Remember that your purpose is to get your teen to open up — not shut down as a result of you dominating the conversation.

- *"Between 1–10 (10 = highest), how would you rate your personal relationship with the Lord?"*

- *"Do you think that being a Christian makes a difference in your life? Why, or why not?"*

- *"What kinds of pressures do teenagers like yourself face concerning the use of alcohol? drugs? smoking? chewing? How do you handle these pressures?"*

- *"Do you feel a sense of purpose or destiny for your life? What might that be?"*

- *"In five years, do you see yourself still serving the Lord? Is there anything in your mind right now that might prevent you from wanting to serve the Lord in the future?"*

- *"Between 1–10 (10 = highest), how would you rate your relationship with your parents?"*

- *"Between 1–10 (10 = highest), how would you rate your relationship with your friends?"*

- *"What are the five things you value most in life? Why?"*

- *"Do you feel you can safely share your true feelings with your parents, i.e., without being judged or condemned?"*

- *"If you had a close friend who was using drugs or alcohol, what would you tell him? How would you act around him? Would you continue to love and support him?"*

- *"What feelings do you have about life when you are all alone? Are your feelings when you're all alone different from the feelings that you have when you're with your family? with your friends?"*

- *"If you were to draw a picture that described how your life is right now, what would the picture look like? What would make it look this way?"*

- *"If you could change anything about your life, what would you change?"*

## 4 Take Action

The goal of this section of *The Parent Connection* is not to alarm or frighten you about your teen. If this chapter causes only one family to notice signs of alcohol or drug involvement in its teen(s), then it has served its purpose.

❑ After reading this section and talking with your teen, do you feel your teen needs professional help for drug or alcohol use? Yes / No / I don't know

❑ Do you feel that you need to contact Al-Anon (a group that supports families and friends of alcoholics) to help you deal with your feelings toward your teen? Yes / No / I don't know

❑ Do you want to contact the youth pastor at your church about your teen's substance abuse problem? Yes / No / I don't know

❑ Do you want to have a serious talk with your spouse about what your next step should be concerning your teen's conflict? Yes / No / I don't know

❑ Do you feel that you have a good support group in your extended families that would help you? Yes / No / I don't know

❑ If you know that your teen isn't involved with drugs or alcohol, are you still concerned about his possible tobacco use? Yes / No / I don't know

❑ Do you and your spouse feel that you need to plan a specific time alone with your teen to confront him about his possible use of alcohol, drugs, or tobacco? If so, fill in the following concerning that meeting:

date:_____

time: _____

location:_____

attendees:_____

subject:_____

procedure: _____

❑ Do you feel that you would like to talk to a close friend about this issue before you draw any conclusions? Yes / No / I don't know

If so, the name of the person is:_____

I will call him/her:_____

## *5* Pause to Reflect

After finishing the appropriate Action Steps, use the following questions to evaluate your session with your teen so that the next one can be even better.

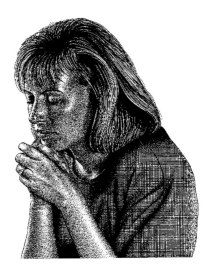

● After trying the Action Steps, how do you feel?

Worried about your teen

Challenged to talk with your teen

Confident that your teen is okay

- How well did you "connect" with your teen on this issue? Why or why not?

  Not very well     Fairly well     Very well

- How well did the Conversation Starters work with your teen on this topic?

  Not very well     Fairly well     Very well

- Did you learn anything new about your teen that you didn't know before you went through this section? If so, what did you learn?



- Did you learn anything new about yourself that you didn't know before you read this section? If so, what did you learn?



- Will you try to believe and apply the three C's of Al-Anon to your situation with your teen?

  "I didn't cause it." Personal application:_____
  _____

  "I cannot cure it." Personal application:_____
  _____

  "I cannot control it." Personal application:_____
  _____

- While you were reading this section, did you become concerned about another person(s) — besides your teen — who may have a problem in this area? If so, record the name(s) below. Begin to pray for this person(s), asking the Lord how He might want you to proceed.

  The name of the person(s):_____
  _____

- Record any further insights, questions, or comments about your teen and this section here:

## Further Resources

Look up your local Al-Anon or Alcoholics Anonymous chapter in your phone book.

*Masquerade, Unveiling Our Deadly Dance With Drugs and Alcohol*, Milton Creagh, Focus on the Family.

*God Is For The Alcoholic*, Jerry Dunn, Moody Press, 1986.

*The Twelve Steps for Christians*, RPI Publications, 1994.

*The Life of the Party: A True Story of Teenage Alcoholism*, Becky Tirabassi with Gregg Lewis, Campus Life Books, Zondervan, 1990.

# SPIRITUAL HEALTH

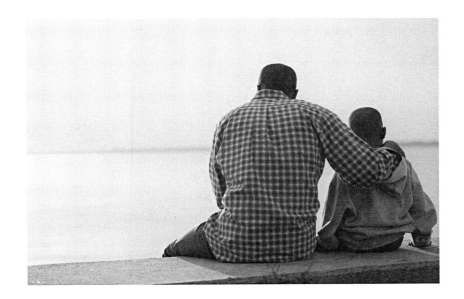

*Children will tend to experience seasons of ebb and flow in their pursuit of God. The question to ask ourselves is not, "Is my child as spiritually mature as I would like?" but, "Is my child more spiritually mature than at this point last year?" As they grow spiritually, their appetite for God should increase. If not, we must look for evidence of sickness in their relationship with Him.*[74]

# CHAPTER TWENTY-THREE

# Teens Riding the Spiritual Fence

When I was in seventh grade, I went forward and gave my life to Christ at a Christian concert. I knew that something had happened. I felt a sense of newness come to my life. I had a great desire to read the Bible and pray. As time passed, however, I had no one to talk with about my "new life" in Christ. Consequently, I began to doubt the validity of what had happened at the concert. The good feelings began to dwindle. Since I didn't "feel" like a Christian anymore, I concluded that I wasn't.

During the next four years, I responded to similar salvation messages seven separate times. No one told me that I wouldn't always "feel" like a Christian. No one informed me that becoming a Christian did not exempt me from trials and temptations. As a result, whenever I failed or experienced intense temptation, I thought that I had to give my life to Christ all over again. It wasn't until I was a high school junior that someone noticed my doubting and inability to get "spiritually" moving. They pointed out to me that I had been sitting on a spiritual fence for four years and had been unable to be spiritually productive because I had been living by feelings instead of by faith. To overcome my wavering once and for all, I set a date for my salvation and recommitted my life to Jesus Christ. At that moment, I determined to walk by faith and not by emotions. I realized that my position in God, as His adopted child, had never changed since the first time I prayed to receive Jesus. I put my total trust in God and focused my full attention on my spiritual future. I stopped depending on my own ability to live "right."

> "Our perseverance during apathetic seasons should have, as its goal, to teach our children to live by faith and not by their feelings. Like us, they will not always *feel* God's presence. They may not *feel* like participating in worship. We can be tempted at such times to entertain anxious thoughts about their relationship with the Lord, to lecture them or to give in to their desire to curtail their

involvement in the church. Such reactions are usually motivated by fear and only accentuate their tendency to live by how they are feeling." [75]

A spiritual "fence" is a position of neutrality or indecision. It separates two distinct property lines. Is your teen having a hard time deciding whether or not to serve God? He may seem to "act" spiritual, but do you doubt his personal relationship with God? Is your teen obviously disinterested in spiritual things? Does she frequently respond in surprising — if not shocking — ways? Sometimes teens step out from under their parent's spiritual umbrella to see what it's like not to be "spiritual." At other times, their lukewarmness can be a time of simple curiosity or, more seriously, a display of open rebellion. I have heard teens say, "Once I graduate from this school...." or, "Once I'm able to move out of my parent's house, I'm going to do whatever I want to do." Whatever the verbal expression, your teen may be riding the spiritual fence. It's never too late to influence his decision for God. Getting a teen off of his spiritual fence requires much love, acceptance, honesty, perseverance, forgiveness, and prayer.

# 1  Know the Causes

Teens hop on the spiritual fence most often as a result of the following factors:

- negative influences (peers, media, music, entertainment)
- disillusionment with God, the church, or Christianity in general
- having no sense of divine vision or destiny
- a time of self-reflection and owning his/her own faith
- being spiritually abused; seeing a loved one get spiritually abused; being forced to serve God
- observing hypocrisy in their family, youth group, friends, or church

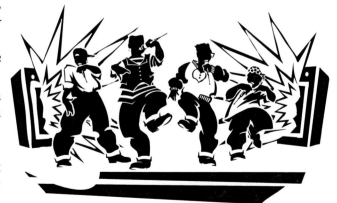

Let's look more closely at several of the above causes.

### Negative influences (peers, media, music, entertainment)

Teens on the spiritual fence pay more attention to the negative influences from which their parents have tried to keep them away. They seem to listen more to what their peers say than taking their parent's input or advice. Their desire for worldly things becomes clear, and their habits and activities change. Teens may withdraw from their families and isolate themselves. It takes alert parents to notice the sometimes subtle changes in their teen's spiritual life.

### Disillusionment with God, the church, or Christianity in general

A season of disenchantment with God, the church, or Christianity in general is common among young people. Adults often experience the same symptoms: "Does God really hear me when I pray?," "God seems so far away from me." All the truths that teens have been taught about God are questioned. Teens sometimes question their own position in Christ, "How do I know for sure that God really loves me?" Teens can also become disillusioned as they overhear their parents complain about their church and its leadership. If a church staff person hurts a family member or close friend, teens will generally have a more difficult time forgiving and moving on than their parents. Parents need to evaluate closely whether a certain season of disillusionment can be resolved through the forgiving of offenses or whether it's the beginning of a serious spiritual decline.

### Having no sense of divine vision or destiny

When teenagers have no purpose in their lives, a sense of spiritual apathy and aimlessness sets in. Parents can easily mislabel such apathy as laziness or rebellion, when actually their teens simply need God to plant within them a keen awareness of His destiny for their life.

### A time of self-reflection and owning his own faith

This can also be a time when teens may be subconsciously shedding the skin of their parent's faith and beginning to "own" their own. Teens may ask themselves inside, "Do I believe in God because my parents do, or because I really believe in God?" "Do I want to serve God because my parents want me to, or because I want to serve Him?" This shifting of ownership of faith is a healthy and an important process. It doesn't happen overnight, and it's very necessary for a teen's mental and emotional maturity. It takes a very discerning parent to know the reason why his teen seems to be in a season of indecision.

## 2 Observe Your Teen

The following observations will help you to notice if your teen is riding the spiritual fence.

- Does your teen seem to "act" spiritual much of the time but lack his own genuine relationship with God? Yes / No / I don't know

- Has your teen been focusing more of his attention on worldly influences (i.e., unhealthy music, on-the-edge movies, non-Christian books) rather than on more spiritual activities? Yes / No / I don't know

- Does your teen often refer to "not feeling" like going to church or spiritual functions? Yes / No / I don't know

- Do your teen's friends, for the most part, have non-Christian values?
  Yes / No / I don't know

- Has your teen asked questions about God and Christianity that make you think that he's doubting his own salvation?
  Yes / No / I don't know

- Has your teen been making statements about God and Christianity that make you think that he's questioning whether he wants to serve God? Yes / No / I don't know

- To your knowledge, how often does your teen read his Bible?
  Infrequently    Semi-frequently    Frequently

- Has your teen made negative remarks about your church or church leadership that make you believe that he may be carrying an offense?
  Yes / No / I don't know

- Do you believe that your teen inwardly resents you because you have been so strict? Yes / No / I don't know

- Do you believe that your teen inwardly resents you because of all the time that you spend at church functions? Yes / No / I don't know

- Can you see negative attitudes in your teen now that you didn't address in his early childhood? If so, what are some of these attitudes?

  Yes / No / I don't know

  Negative attitudes: _____

- Has your teen experienced a major disappointment that you believe is negatively affecting his/her relationship with God? If so, what was the disappointment and how is your teen choosing to respond to it?

  Yes / No / I don't know

  Disappointment and response: _____

## 3 Talk with Your Teen

When parents watch their teens experience a season of spiritual apathy — even serious rebellion — they pause to reflect. Some of the questions that begin to bombard parents' minds are: "Where did we do wrong?" "What can we do to help our teen make the right choices?" "Were we too harsh when he was growing up?" In order to avoid unnecessary guilt and condemnation during such times, I recommend that parents do the following:

- Pray to God to show you any areas for which you need to apologize to your teen. If you have been too harsh, judgmental, legalistic, or forceful, asking his forgiveness (and expecting nothing in return) could turn your child totally around. If you feel that you need more insight into the matter, go to a qualified Christian family counselor.

- If, after reflective prayer and counsel, you and your spouse don't see that you have anything for which to ask your teen forgiveness, ask your teen whether she feels that you have hurt or offended her directly. In order for your teen to respond truthfully when you ask her whether you have deeply hurt or offended her, she must sense that you are totally humble and sincere. She must feel that your question is not just another opportunity that you have created in order to "lecture" her about better serving God. Wait for the correct, undistracted moment to bring the subject up to your teen, and then do a lot of listening. Don't put words into your teen's mouth, but have a few questions ready if necessary. E.g., "Have you felt that we have ever been too: harsh, strict, closed-minded, judgmental, rigid, rejecting, forceful, etc.?"

It's totally normal for parents to have self-reflective questions and doubts when their teen is experiencing a spiritual crisis. But, it's vitally important that each parent has within himself the knowledge that his teen has his own free will. Your teen is making his own choices. Don't punish yourself unnecessarily for being a "bad" parent. You cannot control your teen's choices. However, you can pray for him to have wisdom and strength to make the right decisions. You can stay connected with him and give input whenever you can throughout the whole process. Don't give up. Parents and church leaders can teach teens how to seek God, read their Bibles, and worship; but, unless a teen applies what he has learned, it doesn't amount to anything but intellectual knowledge.

A teen can choose to become a perpetual observer and never go out and apply the knowledge, faith, and wisdom he has learned. Teens need to be reminded of the "How to's" of the Christian walk, but they need — even more — to be led into a personal relationship with Jesus which is continually growing. How can we help our teens to reach out to God and get to know Him more and more personally? To more spiritually sensitive teens, it might work to ask, "When you meet with the Lord, will He know you as an intimate friend or a casual acquaintance?" But, to those teens who are struggling, parents need to try to ascertain their teen's point of struggle and respond wisely and sensitively. Some of teenager's most common spiritual frustrations are:

- "Why should I pray?"

- "What should I do? The Bible seems so boring to me."

- "How do I know God hears me when I pray?"

- "I don't know what to say to God."

- "What if I'm mad at God?"

- "What if I don't have time to pray or read the Bible?"

- "What if I've sinned?"

- "What if I don't feel like praying?"

- "What if I'm distracted or want to go to sleep during prayer?"

- "Do I have to go to church to be a Christian?"

- "Is God going to judge me if I don't obey all of our church's rules and regulations?"

- "What if I don't think that God will answer me when I pray?"

- "What if I don't think God cares about me and my problems?"

After reading all of the following questions, choose which ones would be the most effective ways for you to use to begin a casual conversation with your teen. Remember that your purpose is to get your teen to open up — not shut down as a result of you dominating the conversation.

- *"Do you ever feel like God is far away? How does this make you feel?"*

- *"Do you ever wish you were not a Christian?"*

- *"Do you think being a Christian is fun? What does it mean to have fun?"*

- *"Do you think that the Bible has the answers for life's problems?"*

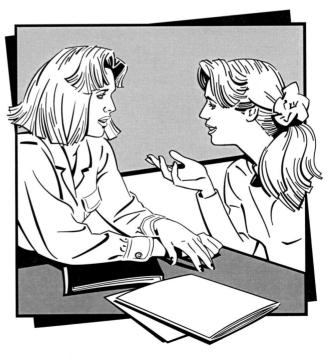

- *"Do you think God can speak to you personally through the Bible? Has He ever spoken to you this way?"*

- *"How do you think God speaks to His people these days?"*

- *"Do you think a person can really feel the presence of God? Have you ever felt Him? What does His presence feel like to you? Do you think it's the same for everyone? Why or why not?"*

- *"What does it mean to walk by faith and not by feelings? How can teenagers as well as adults do this?"*

- *"Do you feel that you've had a personal encounter with Jesus? Have you made Him the Lord of your life?"*

- *"What do you think it means to make Jesus the Lord of your life?"*

- *"Do you ever feel like giving up on your Christian walk? What makes you feel this way? What do you do when you feel this way?"*

- *"What does it mean to persevere? How does this apply to your walk with God?"*

- *"Do you ever find yourself comparing your "spirituality" with that of your peers? In what ways do you compare yourself? How do you know the true condition of their relationship with God?"*

- *"Have you ever been disappointed with God? What made you disappointed? How did it make you feel? Did it affect your daily relationship with Him?"*

- *"What are some of the signs that a teenager may be doubting his faith?"*

## 4 Take Action

The goal of this section is to help you to "connect" with your teen on a spiritual level. The spiritual level on which you find that you connect with your teen may not be your spiritual level or even the level you had hoped for in your teen. The point is to connect wherever he is at without being disappointed and without lecturing. You need to show the same grace to your teen that God shows to you every day.

You can use the following Action Steps to bring more practicality to your spiritual connection with your teen.

❏ After reading this section and talking with your teen, how have you found your teen's spiritual health to be?

Lower than what I expected     About where I expected     Better than I expected

❏ Do you believe that your teen is riding the spiritual fence? If so, rank the following options in the order that you feel has influenced her to do so (1 = the most influential; 6 = the least influential)

_____ negative influences (peers, media, music, entertainment)

_____ disillusionment with God, the church, or Christianity in general

_____ having no sense of divine vision or destiny

_____ a time of self-reflection and owning her own faith

_____ experiencing or observing spiritual abuse; being forced to serve God

_____ observing hypocrisy in their family, youth group, friends, or church

❏ After reading this section and talking with your teen, with whom do you plan to talk about your teen's spiritual life?

_____ your teen's youth pastor

_____ a close friend

_____ your pastor

_____ a professional Christian counselor

❏ Do you believe that your teen needs more spiritual input from you and your spouse right now? Yes / No / I don't know

❏ If your answer to the last question was "yes," how will you give him more spiritual input?

_____ through a better example; work on your own spiritual life

_____ start using a daily or weekly devotional with him

_____ improve your present family devotions

_____ show more grace to your teen instead of legalism and law

_____ do more fun things with him to deepen your relationship

_____ other:_____

❑ Do you plan to talk with your spouse about your teen's spiritual health? If so, when? Yes / No / I don't know

When: _____

##  5 Pause to Reflect

After you finish the Action Steps that you believe will work the best for you, you can benefit from evaluating how well this material worked with your teen so that the next section might work even better.

- After reading this section and doing some of the Action Steps, are you concerned about your teen's spiritual health?

  Yes / No / I don't know

- How well did you "connect" with your teen in this section?

  Not very well      Fairly well      Very well

- How well did this section's Conversation Starters work with your teen?

  Not very well      Fairly well      Very well

- What did you learn about your teen from this section that you didn't know before reading this section?

- What did you learn about yourself — and your parenting style — that you didn't know before reading this section?

- Is your own relationship with the Lord growing and deepening? Explain.


- Can your teen see visible evidence in your home of your growing relationship with God, i.e., your increasing hunger, love, zeal, service, etc.? Explain.


- Record any further insights, questions, or comments about your teen's spiritual health here:


## Further Resources

*Raising Kids Who Hunger For God*, Benny & Sheree Phillips, Chosen Books, 1991.

*Extreme Faith. Freedom in Christ for Teens.* Neil Anderson and Dave Park, Harvest House, 1996.

*Student Prayer Journal*, Becky Tirabassi, Thomas Nelson, 1991.

*40 Days with God, A Devotional Journey.* Rebecca St. James, Empowered Youth Products, 1996. CD ROM included.

*Decision Making and the Will of God*, Garry Friesen, Multnomah Press, 1967.

# CHAPTER TWENTY-FOUR

# The Need for Spiritual Vision

*Our generation needs a fresh understanding of [their] purpose – where they came from, where they're going, and why in the world they're here!* [76]

When I was a teenager, no one talked to me about having a divine destiny. I tried hard to do what was right, but, for a long time, I didn't seem to have great success living the Christian life. When the time came that I had to decide what college to attend, I knew that the Lord wanted me to seek Him to discover His will in the matter. When I began to seek God about where to go, a deep sense of purpose began to develop inside of me — even though I didn't have an exact picture of what I was going to do. As that sense of destiny stayed with me, it gave me the strength I needed to withstand temptation.

Pastor Wendell Smith explains it this way: "The greatest deterrent to sin is not religious rules — but vision!"[77] "Without a vision, the people perish." says Proverbs 29:18. Teenagers desperately need their own fresh vision; a motivating cause given to them by God which gives them a purpose for living. Generally, teens lack motivation about many things: academics, family, relationships, planning for the future, and, unfortunately, their relationship with God. Those teens, however, who personally experience God and continue to receive fresh vision from Him, have a special drive and motivation that infects every area of their lives. I have seen it repeatedly: the teens who have vision are much less likely to sin or backslide. Why? Because they know that every detour will hinder them from fulfilling their divine destiny. Do you know whether your teen has a deep sense of purpose? If your teen doesn't, how can you help him obtain one?

# 1 Know the Causes

What makes one teen have a sense of destiny and another not? I've observed that the more of the following factors that a teen has operating in his life, the more he tends to have a divine vision and purpose for living and the future.

- gives God many opportunities to speak to him

- is around positive peers who are seeking the same things

- has a strong youth leader who trains him on how to seek God

- meditates in the Word of God

- prays by himself and with others

- has parents and family who share about what God is doing all over the world

- has parents who challenge him to be in "hot pursuit" of God's purpose

- has parents who pray for him to sense a strong personal destiny in God

Teens can also catch a vision for their lives in an instant: at church camp, during a counseling session, hearing the testimony of a missionary, listening to a tape, watching a ministry video, meditating in Scripture, etc. The most important contribution you can make as a parent, along with praying for your teen, is to allow God as many opportunities as possible to speak to and touch your teen. That means going to church regularly, encouraging family and private devotions, and attending special ministry meetings that might come to town.

It's ultimately up to your teen to hear and respond to what God says to him inside. You can help the process along by giving your teen opportunities to discuss openly the desires he already has deep within. Many teens think that to receive a vision from God they must be translated to a "higher plane" and be given a complete picture in their mind of all they will ever do for God. This, realistically, is not usually the way God works. His vision or destiny for a teen can come as simply and quietly as a desire in the heart to be a teacher, doctor, missionary, etc. Destiny can be seen in a great talent or skill that your teen has developed and really enjoys. Whatever your teen's unique situation, you can help the most by motivating him to seek more of God. Remember, seeking a purpose for living means seeking the Creator of that purpose.

## 2 Observe Your Teen

Here are a few important questions to ask yourself about your teen:

- Do you think that your teen lacks a vision for his life?
  Yes / No / I don't know

- Do you think that your teen feels that he has nothing to offer God? Yes / No / I don't know

- Do you think that your teen compares himself with his peers' skills, gifts, and talents? Yes / No / I don't know

- Do you think that your teen compares herself with her peers' spirituality?
  Yes / No / I don't know

- Do you feel that you and your spouse should challenge your teen more to seek God's purpose for his life?
  Yes / No / I don't know

- Does your teen seem apathetic and aimless concerning her life?
  Yes / No / I don't know

- Do you think that your teen is bored with his Christian walk?
  Yes / No / I don't know

- Do your teen's friends seem to be apathetic about life; lacking a sense of vision and destiny? Yes / No / I don't know

- Do you think that your teen is waiting around for "a blast from heaven" to reveal God's vision and destiny to him?

  Yes / No / I don't know

  > "Our goal in life is not to decide what we want to do, but to discover what He has destined us to do!"[78]

As I became more informed about how God has a special vision and destiny for each of us to fulfill, I realized that I've made a couple of mistakes with our five-year-old son, Steven, in talking to him about his destiny. The first mistake I made was that I didn't phrase my question correctly. Instead of leaving the decision up to him by asking him, "What do you want to do when you grow up?," I should have asked him, "What do you think God wants you to do when you grow up?" The fact is that God is the initiator, and teens are the responder. The second mistake I made was trying to influence Steven to do what his Dad and I would like to see him do, i.e., be a preacher, evangelist, doctor, etc.

Too many times I asked Steven, "Wouldn't you ever want to have the job of preaching like our pastor?" "No," he always replies, "it doesn't sound as fun as being a police officer!" The fact is that God's plan for a teen is frequently different than the plan that a teen's parents have for him. At Steven's young age, it's only normal that his desires for the future would change every day. One day he wants to be a fireman, the next day a construction worker, and the next day a police officer. But, eventually, as his Dad and I avail him of many opportunities to hear God's direction for himself, he will find his destiny, be happy, and draw a smile from his heavenly Father.

When a teenager feels that one or both of his parents is disappointed or critical of his interests, it can be very spiritually and emotionally damaging to him. God may be beginning to plant a great dream in him, and we may be hindering its development. During adolescence, teens are trying to find who they are and what they should pursue. One of the best ways for them to do so is to be allowed to follow certain avenues of their own interest, in innocent areas, of course. It's healthy for them is to learn how to come to such conclusions on their own, by trial-and-error, through the joys and sorrows of their own choices. This is how teens get to know themselves and discover what makes them "tick" inside. Teens need to develop their own self-identity — separate from the group mind — and pursuing many different personal interest areas is a safe way for them to start to do it. Through working through their own thoughts and feelings, they can decide whether they want to continue to pursue some direction or not. If Dad and Mom, however, are constantly telling their teen what to think, how to feel, and what to do, then that habit of dependency may continue on into their twenties and beyond.

My brother once worked at a prestigious men's clothing store in our city. One day a father came into the store with his son. The father was about 60 years old, and his son about 35. Both of them wanted to buy their own sport coat outfit. During the course of making their buying decisions, the son capitulated to every one of his father's suggestions — and subtle manipulations — as to what he felt his son should buy. As these two grown men stepped up to the counter to pay for their merchandise, everyone in the store observed that the son ended up purchasing the exact same sport coat, shirt, and slacks as his father purchased for himself! In learning from this father-son relationship, it isn't very difficult to conclude that if this man's father was still controlling his garment buying decisions at the age of 35, his father probably never let his son learn to make his own decisions — especially in his teens. Learning to make their own decisions and learning from their own mistakes, is how teens grow up, find themselves, and become responsible decision-makers.

## 3 Talk with Your Teen

After reading all of the following questions, choose which ones would be the most effective ways for you to use to begin a casual conversation with your teen. Remember that your purpose is to get your teen to open up — not shut down as a result of you dominating the conversation. Keep in mind that your teen might hesitate to share his dreams with you if he feels that you might reject or criticize his feelings or desires.

- *"What do you think it means when a teen says that he has a divine vision for his life?"*

- *"What do you think helped Paul the apostle to endure all of his trials?"*

- *"What do you feel that God wants you to do with your life? What makes you feel that this direction is from the Lord?"*

- *"If a teen doesn't have a vision for his life, how would you suggest that he pursue one?"*

- *"Once a teen senses God's will for his life, how would you suggest he walk it out practically?"*

- *"Do you sometimes feel that God is keeping His purpose for your life a secret? Do you think He wants His purpose to be hard to find? What might be some reasons that some teens don't find their divine destiny when God is so anxious to show them?"*

- *"What are some of the ways that God uses to communicate to teens about their future?"*

- *"Do you perceive yourself, God, parents, friends, or opportunity to be the main source of vision for your life? How might this question relate to some of the reasons that teens can get confused about what to do in life?"*

- *"Why do you think the disciplines of prayer and reading the Word are so difficult for teens to do?"*

- *"Do you think that God usually shows a teen all of His will at once, or provides only small pieces of the puzzle at a time? If small pieces at a time, why do you think God works this way?"*

- *"What teen issues might hinder you from discovering and accomplishing your divine destiny? What can you do to prevent these issues from blocking God's purpose in your life?"*

- *"What does the word 'ministry' mean to you? Who do you consider to be 'in the ministry'? Do you think that the term 'ministry' applies only to those in church-related positions like pastors, counselors, or missionaries? Do you think that painting contractors, real estate agents, public school teachers, waitresses, etc. can have jobs that are pleasing to the Lord as well as valid 'ministries'? If so, how?"*

# 4 Take Action

The goal of this section is two-fold: first, it's meant to challenge your teen to pursue God's vision for his life through prayer, discussion with significant others, and exposing himself to as many opportunities as possible to hear from God. Second, it's to encourage you actively to support your teen's efforts to fulfill his divine destiny.

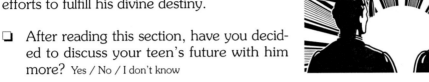

❏ After reading this section, have you decided to discuss your teen's future with him more? Yes / No / I don't know

❏ Will you and your spouse plan a time with your teen to discuss his feelings about the future? Yes / No / I don't know

❏ Will you and your spouse share with your teen your own experiences of how God has led you through the years and/or given you fresh purpose in life? If so, be sure to include whether your experience was progressive or all-at-once. Yes / No / I don't know

❏ Encourage your teen to keep a prayer journal to help her with her daily devotions. In the journal, have your teen record specific prayers, answers to prayers, disappointments, feelings about and questions to God, dreams, visions, and meaningful verses from Scripture.

❏ Explain to your teenager that serving the Lord and having a ministry does not necessarily mean working for a church, being a pastor, or preaching on the mission field. Illustrate for him how *every* Christian serves the Lord in whatever capacity He places them because all of life is sacred to the Lord — not just church life. Tell him that one of the joys of the Christian life is to discover one's spiritual gifts and then to use them in whatever one's circle of influence is. Wherever they are, Christians are to do their work enthusiastically for God and not for men.

❏ To assist your teen in his quest for divine purpose, you can: (1) contact career counseling resources at your local community college and/or in the Yellow

Pages (2) contact the academic counseling depart-
ments in your local community college or univer-
sity (3) obtain information on how to discover
one's spiritual gifts from your local
Christian bookstore or Christian col-
lege/seminary.

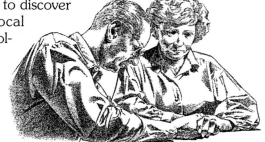

❑ Consistently pray for your teen
that the Lord would give him a
fresh vision for his life.

## 5 Pause to Reflect

After you complete the Action Steps appropriate to your situation, use the following questions to make the next "connection" with your teen even better than the
last one.

● How well did you "connect" with your teen in this section?
Not very well     Fairly well     Very well

● How well did the Conversation Starters in this section work with your teen?
Not very well     Fairly well             Very well

● What did you learn through this material about your teen that you didn't know
before reading this section?

● As a result of going through this section, what did you learn about yourself?

● Do both you and your spouse feel that you are personally fulfilling your divine
destinies? If not, what do you want to do about it?

- Do you feel the need for God to expand the vision that you have for your life and/or family? If so, in what areas would you like God's help in expanding it?


- Record further insights, questions, or comments concerning your teen's purpose in life here:


## Further Resources

*Life On The Edge, A Young Adult's Guide To a Meaningful Life,* Dr. James Dobson, Word Publishing, 1995.

*Make The Big Time Where You Are*, Frosty Westering, Big Five Productions, 1990.

*The Secret: How to Live with Purpose and with Power*, Bill Bright, Thomas Nelson, 1989.

*Dragon Slayer*, Wendell Smith, Generation Ministries of Bible Temple, 1978.

# CHAPTER TWENTY-FIVE

# Hindrances to Spiritual Pursuit

*We may struggle at times in deciding to do the will of God, but we must come to the place where we trust Him with our lives. If He made us, then He knows what's best for us – and what will bring us the greatest fulfillment.*[79]

Teens face unique hindrances as they try to develop their divine potential. What makes their development so challenging is that they do not have years of knowledge or experience to know how to handle these hindrances. The following are seven common obstacles that can keep a teenager from reaching his potential in Christ:

- youthfulness
- distractions
- borrowing trouble
- disappointments with God
- crossing of the wills
- sin and temptation
- looking for shortcuts

## 1 Know the Causes

### Youthfulness

Even though the Bible says, "Let no one despise your youth, but be an example to the believers in word, in conduct, in love, in spirit, in faith, and in purity (I Timothy 4:12), teens still have a hard time being young. It's not so much that they have it "bad," it's just that if they were older they know that they would gain more respect, freedom, and responsibility. Take physical size for instance. Because some teenagers are "late bloomers," they are smaller and more youthful in appearance. Being a "late bloomer" can decrease a teen's self-confidence. The good news, however, is the fact that just because some teenagers are physically smaller than their peers doesn't have to prevent them from beginning to fulfill their divine destinies.

It's very important for a teen's parents not to judge them by their physical appearance — as their peers do all too often. Instead, teens need their parents to believe that they have access to the same divine power as they do; the "dynamite" of the Holy Spirit! Exercising faith and cultivating a personal relationship with God will release that power for any teen who desires it. From what I've observed, God is dynamically moving on teenagers and setting them on fire for God.

## Distractions

Many teens float along in life in whatever direction the wind is blowing. They let the circumstances of life dictate how they feel and ultimately how they live. When teenagers set their mind to seek God, it goes without saying that difficulties will arise that will try to discourage them. One day they may feel great and in tune with God and the next day they may feel like God is a million miles away. It's not that God has moved, it's that feelings change. Changing feelings can easily distract a teen who has not had much time to develop self-control.

That's why it's important to teach our teen-agers to become "God-focused." Use relevant Bible verses in your home along with positive words of faith to help your teen stay focused on God. Satan wants to use anything and everything to distract teens from seriously pursuing God.

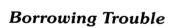

## Borrowing Trouble

My Mom always used to tell me never to "borrow trouble." To "borrow trouble" means to worry about things that you don't even know will come to pass. Bill

Meyer and Dan Zadra relate this to how teens can "borrow trouble" in worrying about losing in athletics:

> "Sometimes we spend so much time thinking about how we might lose, that we forget to think about how we might win. Instead of thinking about how well we're going to do, we spend all of our practice time thinking up imaginary disasters for ourselves." [80]

Does your teenager have the habit of "borrowing trouble?" Does he often think of the bad things that might happen rather than focusing on the positive, promises of God? Remind your teen often that he's on the winning team. If he stays on God's team, he absolutely cannot lose! As a parent, you can help your teen not be so anxious about life by focusing on the positive, speaking encouragement, and sharing the Word of God.

## Disappointments with God

Everyone experiences it, even adults feel it at times. It's the feeling of being disappointed with God. Does your teen ever feel like God is unfair? Does he feel that God ignores him but not others? Has your teen asked the difficult question, "If God loves us so much, why do so many bad things happen?" It's normal for your teen to feel this way – not understanding all of the problems and not understanding God. However, it's what your teen does with his disappointments that will determine how much they could hinder his divine destiny. This is where faith comes into play. Deep trust in God, no matter what the circumstances, is the kind of faith that God wants to develop in your teen. Teach your teenager to "hang in there" and trust God just because He's God, not because he understands the circumstances.

## Crossing of the Wills

Undoubtedly, suffering is part of the Christian package. Sometimes teens begin to experience the pain of conflict even at a young age. Christ said if any one desired to come after Him, they had to deny themselves and take up their cross daily (Luke 9:23). No one is exempt from having to take up the cross and following Christ if he wants to reach his full divine potential. For teenagers, the cross they must bear daily is the inward struggle between their will and God's will. Suffering is saying "no" to self, and saying "yes" to God. Some teens have a harder time with the term "submission" than others. This crossing of the wills is a critical part of teens discovering their destiny in Christ. [81]

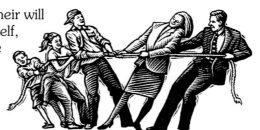

## Sin and Temptation

Dr. James Dobson says that if he could only tell families and young people one thing it would be: "learn to discipline the flesh." If a teenager can learn how to discipline the flesh at a young age, the benefits would follow right into adulthood. Ron Mehl, pastor of Beaverton Foursquare Church, says, "Sin and temptation will always affect your vision." Look at the story of Samson. He had the Spirit of God upon him, and that great power was evident even in his physical strength. Tragically, however, he allowed a lack of discipline of the flesh toward the end of his life to be his downfall. He indulged his own desires rather than resisting them (Judges 16). Can you think of any weaknesses of the flesh that are evident in your teenager?

## Looking For Shortcuts

The best things in life usually require hard work, discipline, and a healthy investment of time. I used to ask my Mother how to spell words as I was doing my homework. "Look that up in the dictionary for yourself," would always be her reply. I didn't feel like taking the large, family dictionary down off the shelf and spreading it all over my work area — I wanted a shortcut. When I taught math class, I observed how teens always wanted a shortcut. They desired to hurry to the end of the problem or look in the back of their textbook for the answers rather than to go through the process of discovering the answer for themselves. We live in a society that wants instant results — the faster and easier the better. Philip Yancey commented, "Shortcuts usually lead away from growth, not toward it." [82]

After His heavenly Father showed Jesus that His ministry was that of a suffering Messiah, Satan tempted Jesus with several shortcuts to His ministry (Matthew 4). The enemy's shortcuts were tempting to Jesus because they would have quickly attracted the masses with a public demonstration of His ability to perform signs and wonders, eliminated His need of daily dependence upon the Father, and circumvented His need to suffer and die. Fortunately for all of us, Jesus refused to take the shortcuts. Encourage your teenager to learn patience and perseverance. Train him not to grow weary while doing what is right (Galatians 6:9). Remember the words of Charles Spurgeon, "Through sheer perseverance, the snail reached the ark!"

# 2 Observe Your Teen

Let's apply these principles to what you've observed in your own teen's life.

- Rank the seven areas below according to how you think they're presently hindering your teen from reaching his full spiritual potential. (1 = the least hindering; 7 = the most hindering)

  \_\_\_\_\_ youthfulness
  \_\_\_\_\_ distractions
  \_\_\_\_\_ borrowing trouble
  \_\_\_\_\_ disappointments with God
  \_\_\_\_\_ crossing of the wills
  \_\_\_\_\_ sin and temptation
  \_\_\_\_\_ looking for shortcuts

- Besides the hindrances listed above, do you think that your teenager has other factors that could hinder her from reaching her spiritual potential? If so, what are they? Yes / No / I don't know

  The other factors: _____

  _____

- List any strengths you see in your teen that he may not see in himself:

- List any weaknesses you see in your teen that she may not see in herself:

- Does your teen, as far as you can tell, have a goal or vision for his life?

  Yes / No / I plan to ask

- Name a significant Christian "other" in your teen's life who might positively motivate your teen to seek God for herself:

It's difficult to talk to someone else about our weaknesses, isn't it? When we do talk about them, though, it can really help. Similarly, if this chapter has shown you a certain weakness in your teen with which you desire to help him, bring it up gently. You may want to do the activity in which both you and your teen record your strengths in one column and your weaknesses in the other column on a clean sheet of paper. By doing this activity along with your teen and demonstrating that you are open to discussing your weaknesses, you should encourage him to open up and discuss his. Discuss with your teen the personal benefit of being aware of our weaknesses: it prevents us from making mistakes. We know what we need to avoid. E.g., if you were on a very strict diet, being aware of the fact that chocolate was one of your major weaknesses, would help you from not going into the chocolate candy store!

## 3  Talk with Your Teen

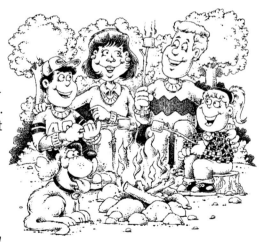

After reading all of the following questions, choose which ones would be the most effective ways for you to use to begin a casual conversation with your teen. Remember that your purpose is to get your teen to open up — not shut down as a result of you dominating the conversation.

- *"Do you ever feel that your age hinders you in any way? Do you feel that it hinders your spiritual growth?"*

- *"Are you looking forward to adulthood? Why?"*

- *"What distractions might keep a teenager from serving God? How can a teenager handle these distractions?"*

- *"Have you ever felt disappointed with God? How have you handled it?"*

- *"What do you think it means to 'pick up our cross daily' and follow Him? What would be an example of a cross you might have to bear?"*

- *"Do you ever feel that you and God are arguing over something? Do you think that God always wins?"*

- *"Do you feel you can totally surrender to God's will and trust Him with your life? What might that mean practically for you?"*

- *"Do you ever fear yielding to sin or temptation? What scares you the most? How do you think you might overcome temptation?"*

- *"Do you find yourself worrying a lot about things that are beyond your own control or that may not even happen? Can you think of an example? How do you usually handle your anxiety?"*

- *"Do you often feel impatient with things or with people? Can you think of an example? Do you think that impatience can hinder a teen from reaching his full spiritual potential? If so, how?"*

## 4 Take Action

The goal of this section is to assist you in identifying some of the ways your teen might be hindered from reaching his divine potential. Through identifying some of his weaknesses, you will be better equipped to help him subdue the enemy. Use the Action Steps below to aid your teen in his spiritual pursuits.

❏ After you read this section, do you want to work with your teen to encourage him to be more positive and optimistic in his outlook on life?

Yes / No / I don't know

❏ Encourage your teen to keep a prayer journal for her daily devotions. In the journal, have your teen record prayers, answers to prayers, disappointments, frustrations, dreams, visions, strengths, weaknesses, spiritual lessons, what the Spirit says to her, and meaningful scriptures. If you were able to do a prayer journal along with your teen, that would be even more exciting for her. Even though you couldn't share everything in your journal with your teen, you could share the safe highlights and she would be thrilled. (see journal sources in the Further Resources section following)

❏ Will you plan on discussing with your teen some of the potential hindrances that he may encounter in the Christian walk? Yes / No / I don't know

❏ Will you talk with your teen about how applying the principle of accountability to his life may help to keep him from taking unnecessary spiritual detours? Yes / No / I don't know

❏ Read the seven common hindrances in this section with your teenager. Ask your teen what she feels might be her greatest hindrance. If it's appropriate, show her how you placed the numbers on the list as you thought of her. You could also perform this exercise on yourself.

## 5 Pause to Reflect

Reflect on how this section affected your teen by answering the questions below.

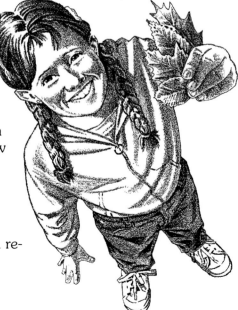

● How well did you "connect" with your teen in this section?

Not very well      Fairly well      Very well

● How well did the Conversation Starters work with your teen?

Not very well      Fairly well      Very well

● What did you learn about your teen from this material that you didn't know before reading this section?

● What did you learn about yourself as a result of doing this section?

- What areas might be hindering you from pursuing God and reaching your full potential in Christ?

- Record any further insights, questions, or comments about your teen's spiritual pursuit here:

## Further Resources

*Disappointment With God*, Philip Yancey, Harper Collins, 1988.

*Challenge, 7 Sessions on Discipleship*, Lyman Coleman, Serendipity House, 1994.

*Faith Training, Raising Kids Who Love the Lord*, Joe White, Focus on the Family, 1994.

*The Ragamuffin Gospel, Embracing the Unconditional Love of God*, Brennan Manning, Multnomah Books, 1990.

*The Bondage Breaker: Overcoming Negative Thoughts, Irrational Feelings, Habitual Sins*, Neil Anderson, Harvest House Publishing, 1990.

# Conclusion

No matter how much of *The Parent Connection* you have completed, you have embarked on a journey to "connect" with your teenager. To connect with him in issues relating to his physical, mental, social, and most important, spiritual health. Getting to know the deeper issues behind what makes your son or daughter think, feel, and act the way he/she does is a huge challenge. Don't lose heart and don't despise small beginnings.

*The Parent Connection* should be used many times. As parents we continually evaluate and then re-evaluate the growth and maturity of our children.

*"Behind every good teen is a good Parent Connection!"*

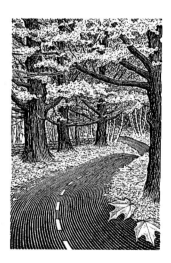

# *The Parent Connection* and the *Total Health* Curriculum

You shall teach these words diligently to your children, and shall talk of them when you sit in your house, when you walk by the way, when you lie down, and when you rise up.

*Deuteronomy 6:7*

## If Your Teen Is Using a Total Health Textbook...

Besides being an excellent stand-alone health resource for parents, *The Parent Connection* can also be easily used along with the *Total Health* series of textbooks (also published by RiversEdge Publishing Co.) which some parents' teens will be using in traditional or homeschool settings. By using *The Parent Connection* in conjunction with your child's *Total Health* textbook, you can more effectively communicate God's principles about health to your teen(s) since you will be more informed. By using the chart below, you can talk with your teen(s) about certain vital health issues in more natural ways (e.g., while driving in the car, at the dinner table, etc.) since you will know what he/she is studying in school.

To use the chart below, find your topic of interest in the first column and, then, in the second and third columns, find the student textbook pages which correspond to it. The second column shows how *The Parent Connection* corresponds with the high school health text (grades 9-12), *Total Health: Choices For A Winning Lifestyle*. The third column shows how *The Parent Connection* corresponds with the middle school health text (grades 6-8), *Total Health: Talking About Life's Changes*.

| The Parent Connection | Total Health: Choices for a Winning Lifestyle (High School) | Total Health: Talking About Life's Changes (Middle School) |
|---|---|---|
| Chapter 1: Nutrition Battles | Chapter 3: Nutrition, pages 61-89 | Chapter 3: Nutrition: Entering the Food Zone, pages 52-69 |
| Chapter 2: Eating Disorders | Chapter 3: Nutrition, pages 90-93 | Chapter 3: Nutrition: What's the Buzz on Dieting? pages 69-77 |
| Chapter 3: Over-exercising | Chapter 4: Fitness & Exercise, pages 97-124 | Chapter 4: Fitness & Exercise, pages 78-95 |
| Chapter 4: Under-exercising | Chapter 4: Fitness & Exercise, pages 97-124 | Chapter 4: Fitness & Exercise, pages 78-95 |
| Chapter 5: Infectious Diseases | Chapter 5: Infectious Disease, pages 125-140 | Chapter 5: Diseases: The Body Under Attack, pages 96-107 |
| Chapter 6: Sexually Transmitted Diseases | Chapter 5: Infectious Disease, pages 140-152 | Chapter 5: Diseases: The Body Under Attack, page 107-108 |
| Chapter 7: Noninfectious Diseases | Chapter 6: Noninfectious Disease, pages 153-178 | Chapter 5: Diseases: The Body Under Attack, pages 108-120 |
| Chapter 8: Reproductive Systems and Human Sexuality | Chapter 2: Eleven Systems: One Body, pages 53-60 | Chapter 2: Human Biology, pages 47-49 |
| Chapter 9: Managing Stress | Chapter 7: Stress & Anxiety, pages 181-192 | Chapter 6: Who Am I? pages 123-130 |
| Chapter 10: Depression | Chapter 7: Stress & Anxiety, pages 192-199 | Chapter 6: Who Am I? pages 139-142 |
| Chapter 11: Developing the Three C's: Conduct, Character, and Convictions | Chapter 8: L.I.F.E. Management, pages 201-211 | Chapter 6: Your Character Counts, pages 134-145; Convictions, pages 108, 233 |
| Chapter 12: Friendships and Peer Pressure | Chapter 8: L.I.F.E. Management, pages 212-215 | Chapter 8: Building Strong Friendships, pages 164-197 |

| The Parent Connection | Total Health: Choices for a Winning Lifestyle (High School) | Total Health: Talking About Life's Changes (Middle School) |
|---|---|---|
| Chapter 13: A Teen's Emotional Earthquakes | Chapter 8: L.I.F.E. Management, pages 215-217 | Chapter 7: Let's Talk About Success: Rebounding from Mistakes, pages 160-162 |
| Chapter 14: The Disciplines of Time Management | Chapter 8: L.I.F.E. Management, pages 218-226 | Chapter 7: Let's Talk About Success: Goal-setting, pages 154-155 |
| Chapter 15: The Issue of Self-Esteem | Chapter 9: Made In His Image, pages 227-238 | Chapter 6: Who Am I?, pages 122-134 |
| Chapter 16: Teens Learning Responsibility | Chapter 12: What's Your Responsibility? pages 299-324 | Chapter 7: Let's Talk About Success, pages 146-159; Chapter 6: Who Am I? Your Character Counts, pages 134-144 |
| Chapter 17: Making Wise Choices | Chapter 13: Maturity: What's It All About? pages 325-333 | Chapter 1: The Power of Choice, pages 2-17 |
| Chapter 18: Abstinence Is More Than Just Saying "NO" To Sex | Chapter 13: Maturity: What's It All About? pages 333-338 | Chapter 8: Building Strong Friendships: Guy/Girl Friendships, pages 180-188 |
| Chapter 19: "Mom and Dad, I'm Pregnant!" | Chapter 13: Maturity: What's It All About? pages 339-342 | (not addressed) |
| Chapter 20: Mixed Messages: Forming Proper Sexual Identity | (not addressed) | (not addressed) |
| Chapter 21: The Dating Game | Chapter 14: Changing Relationships: The Dating Game, pages 359-367 | Chapter 8: Building Strong Friendships: Guy/Girl Friendships, pages 180-188 |
| Chapter 22: Tobacco, Alcohol, and Drugs | Chapter 13: Maturity: What's It All About? pages 343-354 | Chapter 10: Living the Supernatural High, pages 228-266 |
| Chapter 23: Teens Riding The Spiritual Fence | Chapter 15: Building Your Spiritual Muscles, pages 389-410 | Chapter 12: Me, Myself, and God: What Kind of Relationship Do You Have with God? pages 289-298; Will You Count the Cost of Being a Christian? pages 303-305 |

| The Parent Connection | Total Health: Choices for a Winning Lifestyle (High School) | Total Health: Talking About Life's Changes (Middle School) |
|---|---|---|
| Chapter 24: The Need For Spiritual Vision | Chapter 16: Reaching Your Potential, pages 411-415 | Chapter 12: Me, Myself, and God: What's Your View of God? pages 287-289; What Does Your Future Hold? pages 305-311 |
| Chapter 25: Hindrances To Spiritual Pursuit | Chapter 16: Reaching Your Potential, pages 415-423 | Chapter 12: Me, Myself, and God: What Are You Allowing to Influence Your Life? pages 299-302 |

# Notes

1. Josh McDowell, *Right From Wrong*, (Word Publishing, 1994), 125.

2. Ibid.

3. Tim Kimmel, *Raising Kids Who Turn Out Right*, (Multnomah, 1993), 36.

4. Norman W. Walker, *Colon Health: the KEY to a VIBRANT LIFE*, (Norwalk Press, 1979), 1.

5. C. Everett Koop M.D.

6. Cherry Boone O'Neill, *Starving For Attention: A true life story*, (Dell Publishing, 1982), 14-17.

7. James F. Balch, M.D. and Phyllis A. Balch, *Prescription for Nutritional Healing*, (C.N.C. Avery Publishing Group), 92.

8. Minirth, Meier, Hemfelt, Sneed, *Love Hunger: Recovery from Food Addiction*, (Thomas Nelson, 1990), 56-60.

9. Ibid., 55.

10. Michael D.LeBow, *Overweight Teenagers: Don't Bear the Burden Alone*, (Insight Books, 1995), 193-194.

11. Ibid., 185.

12. Ibid., 39.

13. Minirth, Meier, Hemfelt, Sneed, Love Hunger: *Recovery from Food Addiction*, (Thomas Nelson, 1990), 20.

14. Ibid., 43.

15. Michael D. LeBow, *Overweight Teenagers: Don't Bear the Burden Alone*, (Insight Books, 1995), 161.

16. S.I. McMillen, M.D., *None of These Diseases*, (Fleming H. Revell, 1993), 15.

17. *The Healthy Cell Newsletter*, (ALV Publishers).

18. S.I. McMillen, M.D., *None of These Diseases*, (Fleming H. Revell, 1993), 67.

19. Ibid., 58.

20. Dennis and Barbara Rainey, *Teaching Our Children about Sex* Tape Series, (Family Life Today).

21. Dr. James Dobson, *Preparing For Adolescence*, (Regal Books, 1989), 112.

22. Susan Boe, *Total Health: Choices for a Winning Lifestyle*, (RiversEdge Publishing Company, 1995), 153.

23. Dennis and Barbara Rainey, *Teaching Our Children about Sex* Tape Series, (Family Life Today).

24. Ibid.

25. Ibid.

26. Dr. Howard Hendricks, as quoted on, (Family Life Today).

27. James F. Balch, M.D. and Phyllis A. Balch, *Prescription for Nutritional Healing*, (C.N.C. Avery Publishing Group), 270.

28. Ibid.

29. Scott Talley, *Talking with your Kids about the Birds and the Bees*, (Regal Books, 1990), 187-188.

30. Dennis and Barbara Rainey, *Teaching Our Children about Sex Tape Series*, (Family Life Today).

31. Ibid.

32. Jerry White, *Honesty, Morality, and Conscience*, (Navpress, 1983), 218.

33. S.I. McMillen, M.D., *None of These Diseases*, (Fleming H. Revell, 1993), 98.

34. Wendell Smith, *Roots of Character*, (Bible Press, 1979), V.

35. Leo Buscaglia, "*LIFE, There's Nothing Like It*," Pamphlet, (Christopher News Notes, New York, NY).

36. Mike Miller, "*Dare To Live*," Newsletter. Vancouver Washington, 1989.

37. Dr. Mary Griffin and Carol Feisenthal, "*A Cry for Help*" taken from "*LIFE, There's Nothing Like It*," Pamphlet, (Christopher News Notes, New York, NY).

38. Carolyn Kohlenberger and Noel Wescombe, *Raising Wise Children: How To Teach Your Child To Think*, (Multnomah Press, 1990), 26.

39. Ibid., 27-30.

40. Ibid., 30-32.

41. Ibid., 32-33.

42. Howard Ferguson, *The Edge*, a collection of quotes, poems and selections, (Cleveland Ohio: Great Lakes Lithograph Co.), 1.

43. Author Unknown

44. Jerry White, *Honesty, Morality And Conscience*, (Navpress, 1983), 233-235.

45. Ibid., 62.

46. Dr. James Dobson, *Preparing For Adolescence*, (Regal Books, 1989), 60.

47. Dennis Rainey, *Staying Close*, (Word Publishing, 1989), 203.

48. Tim Kimmel, *Raising Kids Who Turn Out Right*, (Multnomah, 1993), 203.

49. Susan Boe, *Total Health: Choices for a Winning Lifestyle*, (RiversEdge Publishing, 1995), 229.

50. Dr. James Dobson, *Preparing For Adolescence*, (Regal Books, 1989), 53.

51. Ibid., 130.

52. Susan Boe, *Total Health*, (RiversEdge Publishing, 1995), 300.

53. Carolyn Kohlenberger and Noel Wescombe, *Raising Wise Children: How To Teach Your Child To Think*, (Multnomah Press, 1990), 12.

54. Ibid., 24.

55. *Help Your Teens Make the Right Choice*, Focus on the Family Newsletter, 1994.

56. Carolyn Kohlenberger and Noel Wescombe, *Raising Wise Children: How To Teach Your Child To Think*, (Multnomah Press, 1990), 24

57. Scott Talley, *Talking with your Kids about the Birds and the Bees*, (Regal Books, 1990), 209.

58. Josh McDowell, *How To Help Your Child Say "NO" To Sexual Pressure*, (Word Publishing, 1987), 40.

59. Scott Talley, *Talking with your Kids about the Birds and the Bees*, (Regal Books, 1990), 166.

60. W.A. Elwall, *Evangelical Dictionary of Theology* ed., (Baker, Grand Rapids, 1984), 422.

61. Scott Talley, *Talking with your Kids about the Birds and the Bees*, (Regal Books, 1990), 169.

62. Josh McDowell, *How To Help Your Child Say "NO" To Sexual Pressure*, (Word Publishing, 1987), 37.

63. Ibid., 40.

64. Dr. James Dobson, *Preparing For Adolescence*, (Regal Books, 1989), 84.

65. Josh McDowell, *How To Help Your Child Say "NO" To Sexual Pressure*, (Word Publishing, 1987), 147.

66. Ibid., 149.

67. Ibid., 151.

68. Dr. James Dobson, *Preparing For Adolescence*, (Regal Books, 1989), 138.

69. Andrew Comiskey, *Pursuing Sexual Wholeness: How Jesus Heals the Homosexual*, (Creation House, 1988), 47-50; 84-87; 89,90.

70. Iverson, Smith, Scheidler, Malmin, *Confronting Our Culture*, (Bible Temple Publishing,) lesson five.

71. Ibid.

72. Benny and Sheree Phillips, *Raising Kids Who Hunger For God*, (Chosen Books, 1991), 56.

73. Ibid., 58-67.

74. Ibid., 245.

75. Ibid., 245.

76. Wendell Smith, *Dragon Slayer*, (Generation Ministries of Bible Temple, 1978), 12.

77. Ibid., 13.

78. Ibid., 15.

79. Ibid., 15.

80. Bill Meyer and Dan Zandra, *The Mental Edge*, an article taken from Sports Motivation Class lecture notes by Frosty Westering.

81. Wendell Smith, *Dragon Slayer*, (Generation Ministries of Bible Temple, 1978), 15.

82. Philip Yancey, *Disappointment with God*, (Harper Collins, 1988), 247.

# Bibliography

Ameiss, Bill and Jane Graver, *Love, Sex & God*. Saint Louis Missouri, Concordia Publishing House, 1988.

Balch, Dr. James F. and Phyllis A. Balch, *Prescription for Nutritional Healing*, C.N.C. Avery Publishing Group.

Boe, Susan, *Total Health, Choices for a Winning Lifestyle*. West Linn, Oregon, RiversEdge Publishing Company, 1995.

Bright, Bill. *The Secret: How to Live With Purpose and Power*. Nashville: Thomas Nelson, 1989.

Buscaglia, Leo, *"LIFE, There's Nothing Like It,"* Pamphlet, (Christopher News Notes, New York, NY).

Capps, Charles, *The Tongue, A Creative Force*. Tulsa Oklahoma, Harrison House, 1976.

Comiskey, Andrew, *Pursuing Sexual Wholeness: How Jesus Heals the Homosexual*. Creation House, 1988.

Dobson, Dr. James. *Preparing for Adolescence*. Ventura: Regal Books a Division of Gospel Light, 1989.

Elwall, W.A., *Evangelical Dictionary of Theology* ed. Grand Rapids, Baker, 1984.

Ferguson, Howard, *The Edge*, a collection of quotes, poems and selections. Cleveland Ohio: Great Lakes Lithograph Co.

Gothard, Bill (instructor). *Institute in Basic Youth Conflicts*. Seminar.

Hales, Dianne, *"How Teenagers See Things,"* Parade Magazine, August 18, 1996.

*"Help Your Teens Make the Right Choice."* Focus on the Family Newsletter, 1994.

Hole, John W Jr. *Human Anatomy and Physiology,* Second Edition. Dubuque, Iowa: Wm. C. Brown Company Publishers, 1981.

Iverson, Dick and Wendell Smith, Bill Scheidler, Ken Malmin. *Confronting Our Culture.* Portland, Oregon: Bible Temple Publishers.

Kidney, Debra. "Dare To Live." *This Week Magazine.*

Kimmel, Tim, *Raising Kids Who Turn Out Right.* Sisters Oregon, Multnomah Books, 1993.

Kohlenberger, Carolyn and Noel Wescombe, *Raising Wise Children, How To Teach Your Child To Think.* Portland, Oregon, Multnomah Press, 1990.

LeBow, Michael D, *Overweight Teenagers, Don't Bear The Burden Alone.* New York, NY, Insight Books, a division of Plenum Publishing, 1995.

*"LIFE There's Nothing Like It."* Christopher News Notes. No. 283.

Malmin, Glenda. *Christian Womanhood*: Course notebook from Portland Bible College, Portland, Oregon.

McDowell, Josh. *How To Help Your Child Say "NO" To Sexual Pressure.* Dallas: Word Publishing, 1987.

McDowell, Josh and Bob Hostetler. "Help Your Teen Make the Right Choice." *Focus on the Family* (November, 1994), 3-4.

McDowell, Josh and Bob Hostetler. *RIGHT FROM WRONG: What You Need To Know To Help Youth Make Right Choices.* Dallas: Word Publishing, 1994.

McMillen, S.I. *None of These Diseases.* Grand Rapids: Fleming H. Revell, division of Baker Book House, 1984.

Miller, Mike. *"Dare To Live."* Newsletter. Vancouver, Washington, 1989.

Minirth, Dr. Frank, Dr. Paul Meier, Dr. Robert Hemfelt & Dr. Sharon Sneed, *Love Hunger, Recovery From Food Addiction*. Nashville, Thomas Nelson Publishers, 1990.

O'Neil, Cherry Boone, *Starving For Attention*. New York, NY, Dell Publishing Company, 1982.

Phillips, Benny and Sheree, *Raising Kids Who Hunger For God*. Grand Rapids Michigan, Chosen Books, 1991.

Pyle, Hugh F, *Sex, Love, & Romance*. Pensacola Florida, A Beka Book, 1989.

Rainey, Dennis and Barbara, *Teaching Our Children about Sex* Tape Series, Family Life Today.

Rainey, Dennis. *Staying Close, Stopping the Natural Drift Toward Isolation In Marriage*. Dallas: Word Publishing, 1989.

Robertson, A.T., *Word Pictures in the New Testament*. Nashville, Broadman Press, 1930.

Ryun, Jim and Anne, *"Courtship Makes a Comeback."* Dobson, Dr. James C, Focus on the Family Magazine, November, 1995.

Smith, Wendell. *Dragon Slayer*. Portland, Oregon: Generation Ministries of Bible Temple, 1978.

Smith, Wendell. *Roots of Character*. Portland, Oregon: Bible Temple Publishing, 1979.

St. Clair, Barry and William H. Jones. *Dynamic Dating*. San Bernardino, California: Here's Life Publishers, 1987.

Talley, Scott. *Talking with Your Kids about the Birds and the Bees*. Ventura: Regal Books, a division of Gospel Light Publications, 1990.

*"The Healthy Cell"* Newsletter, ALV Publishers.

Vredevelt, Pam, *Walking A Thin Line, Anorexia and Bulimia, The Battle Can Be Won*. Portland, Oregon, Multnomah Press, 1985.

Walker, Dr. Norman W., *Colon Health: the KEY to a VIBRANT LIFE*. Prescott Arizona, Norwalk Press, 1979.

Walker, Dr. Norman W. *Pure & Simple Natural Weight Control*. Prescott, Arizona, Norwalk Press, 1981.

Walker, Dr. Norman W, *The Natural Way To Vibrant Health*, Prescott, Arizona, Norwalk Press, 1972.

Walker, Dr. Norman W, *Tune your Mind and Body... Become Younger*. Prescott, Arizona, Norwalk Press, 1972.

*Webster's New Collegiate Dictionary*. Springfield, Mass., Merriam-Webster, 1977.

Westering, Frosty. *Make The Big Time Where You Are!* Big Five Productions. 1990.

Westering, Frosty. *Sports Motivation*. A collection of poems, quotes and personal notations.

White, Jerry. *Honesty, Morality and Conscience*. Colorado Springs: Navpress, 1979.

White, Joe, *Pure Excitement, a radical, righteous approach to sex, love and dating*. Colorado Springs, Colorado, Focus on the Family Publishing, 1996.

Yancey, Philip, *Disappointment with God*. Harper Collins, 1988.

Zandra, Dan and Bill Meyer, *"The Mental Edge,"* an article taken from Sports Motivation Class lecture notes by Frosty Westering.

# NOTES